KV-031-110

The Natural Way Series

Increasing numbers of people worldwide are falling victim to illnesses which modern medicine, for all its technical advances, seems often powerless to prevent – and sometimes actually causes. To help with these so-called 'diseases of civilization' more and more people are turning to 'natural' medicine for an answer. The *Natural Way* series aims to offer clear, practical and reliable guidance to the safest, gentlest and most effective treatments available – and so to give sufferers and their families the information they need to make their own choices about the most suitable treatments.

Special note from the Publisher

The books in this series are intended for information and guidance only. They are not intended to replace professional advice, and readers are strongly urged to consult an experienced practitioner for a proper diagnosis or assessment before trying any of the treatments outlined.

Other titles in the Natural Way *series*

Allergies
Arthritis & Rheumatism
Asthma
Back Pain
Cancer
Chronic Fatigue Syndrome
Colds & Flu
Cystitis
Diabetes
Eczema
Heart Disease
HIV & Aids
Irritable Bowel Syndrome
Migraine
Multiple Sclerosis
Premenstrual Syndrome
Psoriasis

THE NATURAL WAY

Infertility

Belinda Whitworth

Series medical consultants
Dr Peter Albright MD (USA)
& Dr David Peters MD (UK)

Approved by the
AMERICAN HOLISTIC MEDICAL ASSOCIATION
& BRITISH HOLISTIC MEDICAL ASSOCIATION

ELEMENT

Shaftesbury, Dorset • Rockport, Massachusetts
Melbourne, Victoria

© Element Books Limited 1996
Text © Belinda Whitworth 1996

First published in the UK in 1996 by
Element Books Limited
Shaftesbury, Dorset SP7 8BP

Published in the USA in 1996 by
Element Books, Inc.
PO Box 830, Rockport, MA 01966

Published in Australia in 1996 by
Element Books
and distributed by
Penguin Books Australia Limited
487 Maroondah Highway, Ringwood, Victoria 3134

Reissued 1998

All rights reserved.
No part of this book may be reproduced or utilized
in any form or by any means, electronic or mechanical,
without prior permission in writing from the Publisher.

Cover design by Slatter-Anderson
Designed and typeset by Linda Reed and Joss Nizan
Printed and bound in Great Britain

British Library Cataloguing in Publication
data available

Library of Congress Cataloging in Publication Data
Whitworth, Belinda.
Infertility/Belinda Whitworth.
p. cm. -- (The Natural way)
Includes index.
ISBN 1-85230-925-3
1. Infertility–Alternative treatment. 2. Naturopathy.
I. Title II. Series: Natural way series.
RC889.W457 1996
616.6'92–dc20 96–42371
CIP

ISBN 1 85230 925 3

Contents

Illustrations

For Pat

Acknowledgements

Thanks go to all the people who so generously and openly told me about their treatment, to all the practitioners who took the time to tell me about their work, and to all the practitioner and research organizations that answered my queries with such care.

Particular thanks go to Mike Boxhall; Diana Chambers; Beryl Crane of the Reflexology Society; Jenny Dallas; Shelley de Ste Croix; Kris Frank; Lucy Grant and all at the Complementary Health Centre, Exeter; Jean Harris and Lindy Lacey at The Clinic, Tiverton; the Institute of Population Studies, Exeter University; Eve Lane and the Margaret Jackson Centre, Exeter; Duncan McColl; Anne Stobart; Lillian Stoltenberg; Eileen Whatmore at Green Library, London; Helen Gill and the Wyndham House Surgery, Silverton, Exeter.

Introduction

Human fertility is something of a hit and miss affair and infertility is seldom absolute – that is, with zero chance of conception.

The usual figure quoted for couples seeking specialist medical help for infertility is one in six. However, studies have shown that 20 to 35 per cent of people have trouble conceiving at some stage in their lives and that over half of infertile couples do not seek help.

This means that one in three of us could at some stage be going through the worry and misery – often in secret – of wondering whether we'll ever have a child.

Although it is certain that men's sperm counts have dropped dramatically in the last few decades, it is now thought that sperm quality and mobility are more important. It is difficult to say whether we are actually getting less fertile or whether more people are seeking help because more help is available and because we are trying for children later – in our thirties and forties rather than twenties.

Conventional medical intervention can achieve spectacular results. However, the treatments are often lengthy, unpleasant, expensive, not always available, sometimes dangerous or untried and even unnecessary.

Because we do not conceive after a 'normal' period of time, we are driven in panic to seek external help when there is much we can do for ourselves. And in any case, according to the medical profession nearly a third of infertility is 'unexplained'.

Foresight, a British charity set up in 1978 and now with branches worldwide, has had an 81 per cent success rate with its programme of improved diet and lifestyle. When, how and how often you make love may also have a bearing and unfortunately this is not the sort of thing your doctor usually dwells on.

It used to be thought that emotional problems caused 30 to 40 per cent of infertility. That figure is now put at less than 5 and any emotional problems considered the result not the cause. However, it is hard that just when you most need to be happy and healthy circumstances contrive to get you down.

This is where the natural therapies, which treat body, mind and spirit, can give you invaluable support. And not just support. Many have proven success with infertility.

Whatever you decide to do – or not to do – this book aims to give you all the information you need to have the child you want. Good luck.

CHAPTER 1

What is infertility?

How infertility is measured, the things that affect fertility and when to seek help

Infertility means being unable to have a baby when you want one. Like fertility it is a relative term and so it is often difficult to know whether you have a problem or not. One way to judge is against the amount of time it takes other couples to conceive.

Glossary of common terms

fertility	the ability to conceive
infertility	fertility problems
subfertility	the same as 'infertility'
primary infertility	fertility problems in a woman who has never conceived before
secondary infertility	fertility problems in a woman who has conceived before
zero fertility	serious problems such as blocked tubes or lack of sperm which mean a couple can't conceive naturally; congenital problems with reproductive organs
sterility	the same as 'zero fertility'

How long it takes to conceive

A healthy couple in their twenties – the time of peak fertility – can take up to two years to conceive. In their first month of trying a couple has a one in three chance of conceiving and after that it falls quickly to a one in twenty chance each month. This doesn't mean that your fertility falls but that the statistical likelihood of you conceiving gets less. On average, the chance of conceiving each month is 20 to 25 per cent.

Nine out of ten couples in their twenties will have conceived by the end of a year and 95 per cent at the end of two years. This means that, even if there is nothing wrong with you, it can take you over two years to conceive.

Over the age of 30 it can take even longer. One UK survey, for example, showed that three-quarters of women in their thirties took more than two years to conceive.

Age and fertility

The late teens and early to mid twenties are our most fertile years. Before that the reproductive systems in men and women are still developing. Women in their teens may have erratic periods or cycles when they don't ovulate. After their twenties, both men and women start to become less fertile.

Men's fertility declines gradually throughout their lives and women's declines until the menopause around the age of 50 when her monthly cycles come to an end and there is no longer any chance that she can conceive a child. With egg donation and assisted conception techniques, however, she can still bear a child and this is one of the most controversial areas of modern fertility treatment.

Why does fertility decline with age?

Much of our decline in fertility is to do with a general decline in health. The following are examples of this age and health related decline.

- Less efficient blood circulation means that organs work less efficiently. This concerns women particularly since decreased blood circulation to the womb can make it more difficult for an embryo to implant or can make miscarriage more likely.
- More exposure to infection is experienced. Pelvic infection can damage the reproductive organs of both men and women. 'Low-grade' infections – those that have no obvious symptoms so we don't even know we've got them – can change the environment of a woman's body so that the sperm are unable to survive or are upset so that they are less efficient at getting to the egg and fertilizing it.
- More exposure to pollution and radiation can cause abnormalities in the egg or sperm, leading to fertilization failure and miscarriage.

Another possible reason is that people tend to make love less often as they get older.

Women

Women are born with their egg cells so these age as the woman ages. Each month after puberty some of these eggs will start to mature and it is believed that it is the healthiest ones each time that do so. Towards the end of her reproductive years, therefore, a woman may only be left with 'sub-standard' eggs.

Like all the cells in the body, some of the egg cells are dying all the time. The more stress and infection a woman suffers the more egg cells will die, further depleting her store of healthy eggs.

Growths in the ovaries and womb – *cysts* and *fibroids* – are common in all women and increase as women get older. They can distort the organs and stop them working properly.

It is said that women are sterile some ten years before they actually reach the menopause. This is because few women in the past had children over the age of 40 even when newly married. However recent trends would seem to dispute that. According to the UK Office of Population Censuses and Surveys (OPCS), births to women over 40 – although still small in number – increased by over 50 per cent between 1986 and 1996. The OPCS expects this trend to continue.

Women who have already had one or more children are more fertile than those who have never had a child. For example a woman in her late thirties who has had a child may be as fertile as a woman in her early thirties who has not.

Men

The decline in men's fertility is only just being recognized. It is believed that one of the main reasons for the decline is an increase in the number of abnormal sperm. Canadian research in the 1980s showed that at least 16 per cent of sperm from men over 45 have abnormal chromosomes compared with about 4 per cent of sperm from men in their twenties.

Are humans becoming less fertile?

The answer is probably yes, even allowing for the distortion caused by better testing techniques, more treatment being available so more people come forward for treatment, and less reticence about the subject. The reasons may include:

- An increase in sexually transmitted disease because of greater sexual freedom and the use of the contraceptive pill rather than condoms
- Increased pollution and declining nutritional standards
- The fact that we are delaying childbirth till our thirties or even forties

Pollution and nutrition

These are controversial areas but evidence is mounting as to their importance to fertility.

Many scientific studies have shown that pesticides, metals (like lead and cadmium) and chemicals used in industry (such as dioxins produced in the bleaching of paper and polychlorinatedbiphenyls (PCBs) from electronics manufacture) can damage reproduction both in the short term and possibly in the long term (see box on page 6). These pollutants find their way into the water we drink, the air we breathe and the food we eat.

The World Health Organization in its *Guidelines on Diagnosis and Treatment of Infertility* lists exposure to 'harmful environmental agents' as a reason for the decline in fertility of men as they get older. Women with endometriosis (see page 25), the cause of 6 per cent of all infertility, have been found to have higher levels than normal of PCBs in their blood.

Intensive farming and food production techniques mean that our food is much less nutritious than it used to be. Professor Michael Crawford, director of the Institute of Brain Chemistry at Queen Elizabeth Hospital for Children, London, said in 1995 that 'the move to intensive agriculture was the single most important mistake made after the [second world] war. Food has been diluted in terms of nutritional value and accelerated in terms of fats, energy and non-nutritional content.'

A UK government survey in 1991 found that British women between 16 and 49 were deficient in virtually every nutrient and a report on the survey linked this finding with infertility.

Oestrogen mimics and fertility

Scientists are discovering that many modern chemicals such as those in pesticides, plastics and detergents may act on the human body like the female hormone oestrogen.

Oestrogen mimics, as they are known, can affect the baby in the womb and may be responsible for the rise in reproductive birth defects in both men and women. For instance, the incidence of undescended testicles in baby boys has nearly trebled since the 1950s.

They may be the reason that men's sperm counts have dropped 50 per cent since the 1960s because the number of sperm-generating cells men have is fixed before birth.

They may also be behind the growing numbers of women with endometriosis and men and women who have had cancer of the reproductive organs. Testicular cancer has trebled in the last 30 years in both the USA and Britain. Endometriosis has risen from 21 in the world 70 years ago to five million in the USA alone.

Oestrogenic drugs given to women for contraception and as 'hormone replacement therapy' (HRT) may be adding to the problem, not just for the women themselves but because residues of the drugs get into the water supply.

Seeking help

Doctors advise couples under 30 to seek medical help after trying to conceive for two years. Because tests and treatment can take several years, couples over 30 are advised to seek help after a year – even though, as mentioned above, it can take perfectly healthy couples at least two years to conceive, if not longer.

However, the decision as to when or even whether to seek treatment is not a simple one.

Even if doctors find out that you have a problem, they can't always do anything about it. Conventional medical tests and treatment can be stressful and this stress can cause both sperm and ovulation, as well as sexual, problems. On the other hand you may see your fertile years slipping away and feel that nothing is too much trouble.

The natural therapies are almost certain to make you feel better but there is no guarantee that you will receive the outcome you want. They may take time and they are likely to involve you in making changes to your life.

In such a private area as fertility self-help has much to recommend it, but the disadvantage, of course, is that you are alone.

The following chapters should help you judge for yourself whether you may have a problem that needs medical intervention, or whether the natural therapies are more suitable, or whether you would rather continue helping yourself for the moment. Many people find a combination of approaches is the best way of all.

The book starts with a look at the basic workings of a healthy fertile body.

CHAPTER 2

All about the reproductive system

The parts of the body involved in conception and how conception happens

'How pregnancy occurs is remarkably complex', according to Professor (now Lord) Robert Winston of the famous infertility clinic at London's Hammersmith Hospital, and if you go in for conventional treatment you may well be baffled by the array of terms used by doctors. This chapter introduces you to some of them.

Women and reproduction

Women are born with their egg cells or *ova*. These are the largest cells in the body but no bigger than a full stop. They are stored in the *ovaries*, oblong glands about 1½ inches (38mm) long, one each side of the pelvis.

At puberty the ova start to mature, one each 28 days or so. This is the *menstrual cycle*.

Some people think the ovaries take it in turns to mature an egg but in fact the egg can come from either side of the body. If one ovary is damaged or missing the other will take over the entire workload.

Only about 400 ova will mature during a woman's lifetime but she starts out with some two to four million of them.

The reproductive organs and some of the other parts of the body connected with fertility are shown in figure 1 below.

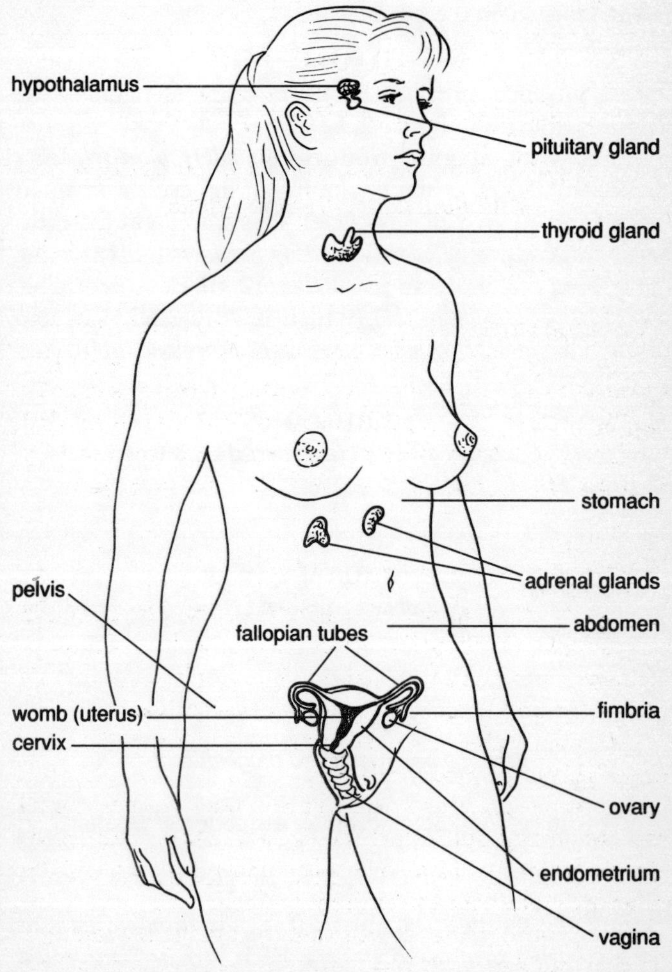

Fig. 1 The reproductive organs in women

The menstrual cycle

The menstrual cycle is run by three glands:

- the *hypothalamus* in the brain
- the *pituitary* in the brain
- the *ovaries*

These produce *hormones*, the chemical messengers of the brain, as shown in figure 2.

The hypothalamus produces *gonadotrophin releasing hormone* (*GNRH*) at the beginning of the cycle and again about day 12 (in a 28 day cycle). This stimulates the pituitary to produce *follicle-stimulating hormone* (*FSH*) for the first part of the cycle until day 12 when it produces *luteinizing hormone* (*LH*) (which is why GNRH is also known as *luteinizing hormone releasing hormone* (*LHRH*)).

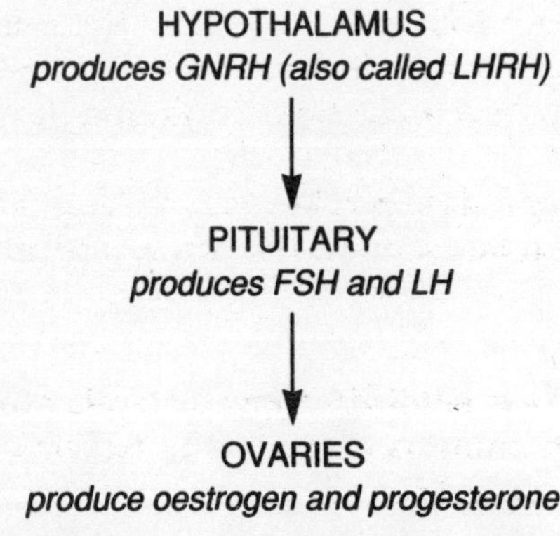

Fig. 2 The reproductive hormone sequence in women

The follicular phase

Stimulated by the FSH, about 20 eggs in the ovaries start to grow and produce *oestrogen*. Each egg is surrounded by a sac called a follicle and so this maturing phase is called the follicular phase.

Ovulation

High levels of LH make the ovaries produce more oestrogen which causes *ovulation*. This is when one of the eggs reaches maturity, bursts out of its follicle and its ovary, is caught (with luck) by the waving fingers or *fimbria* of a *fallopian tube* and starts on its journey to the *uterus* or womb.

By the time of ovulation this 'dominant follicle' will have reached an enormous ¾–1 inch (18–25mm) in size. The other maturing eggs die.

It is thought that about 40 per cent of the time the fimbria of the tube do not manage to catch the egg. However, if one tube is damaged the remaining tube may be able to catch eggs from either ovary.

The luteal phase

The empty follicle left behind in the ovary now starts to produce *progesterone* which makes the lining of the womb or *endometrium* thicken ready for a fertilized egg. Progesterone levels are highest around day 21 of the cycle.

This empty follicle is called the *corpus luteum* ('yellow body') and so this second half of the cycle is called the *luteal phase*.

Menstruation

If the egg is not fertilized hormone levels drop and the extra womb lining is discarded in *menstruation*, also called the *menstrual* period.

The menstrual cycle is shown in figure 3.

Men and reproduction

The reproductive system in men, shown in figure 4, is a complex series of glands and tubes, often referred to by the medical profession as 'plumbing'. Much less is known about it than women's.

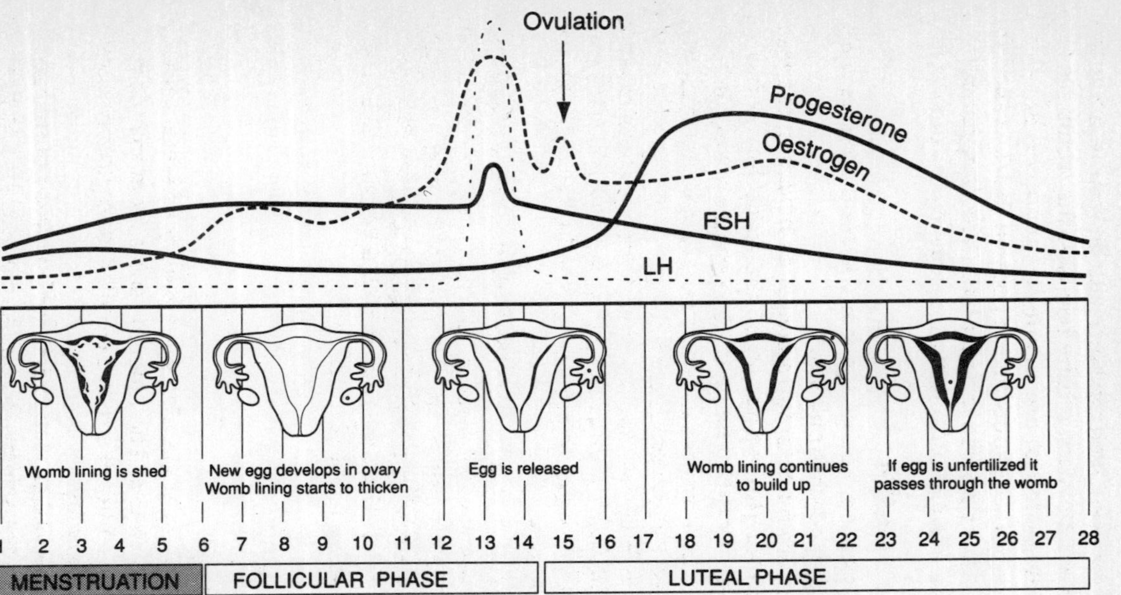

Fig. 3 The menstrual cycle

Like women, men are born with all their reproductive organs intact. When a baby boy is in the womb his two testicles (or *testes*) are inside his abdomen but these 'descend' to hang outside the body in the sac called the *scrotum* shortly before or after birth. This is apparently to keep the organs cool but it also makes them vulnerable.

Sperm production

Spermatozoa, or 'sperm' for short, do not start to be made until a boy reaches puberty.

They are made in the *seminiferous tubules* in the testicles under the influence of the same hormones as women – GNRH, FSH and LH. LH stimulates the testicles to make the male hormone *testosterone* which also influences sperm production.

After about two months, the immature sperm move to the *epididymis*, a mass of tiny coiled tubes, where they continue to mature over the next one to two weeks and are then stored.

Some move on to be stored in the two *vas deferens*, much larger tubes which lead eventually to the penis. These tubes change their name on the way to 'sperm duct' or 'ejaculatory duct' and then join up with the *urethra*, the tube leading from the bladder (the *ureter* is the tube leading to the bladder).

Conception

Ejaculation

In sex the man ejaculates a quantity of *semen* into the woman's *vagina*. The amount varies from man to man but the quantity of a man's ejaculate does not necessarily relate to quality.

Although there are tens if not hundreds of millions of sperm in the semen, they make up only two to five per

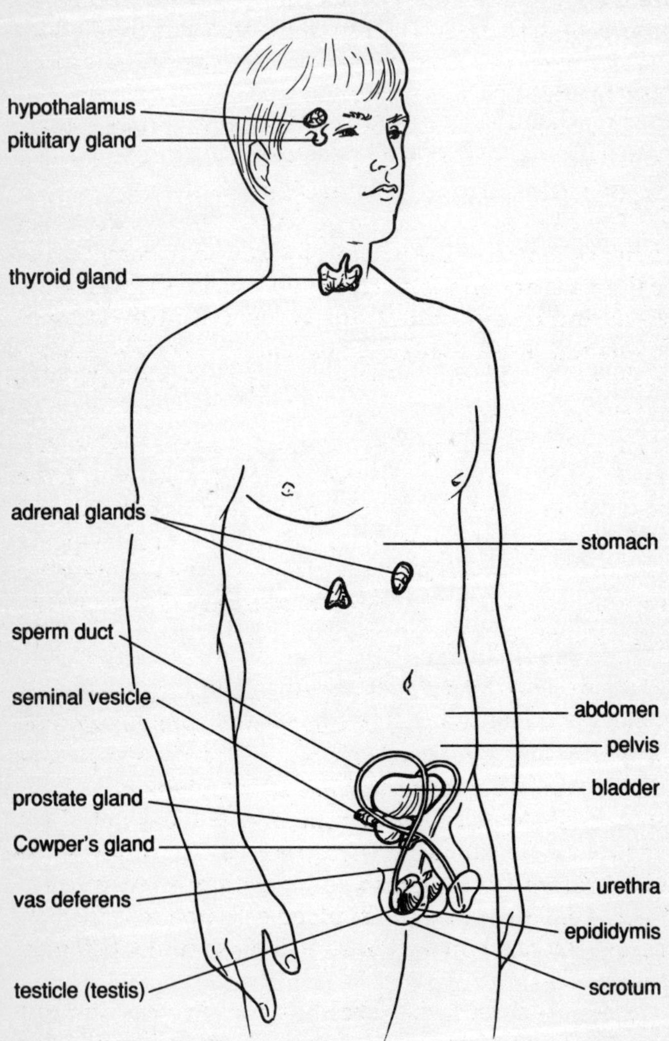

Fig. 4 The reproductive organs in men

cent of it. The amount of sperm in semen can only be checked by analysis. The rest of the semen is fluid which comes from the two *seminal vesicles*, the *prostate gland* and the two *Cowper's glands*.

This fluid contains food for the sperm, protects them and helps transport them. Jelly like to start with, it turns liquid within 20 to 30 minutes of ejaculation.

The vagina is an elastic passage which leads to the *cervix* or mouth of the womb. Normally a woman's internal organs are protected from infection by vaginal secretions and mucus around the cervix but at the time of ovulation these change to become less acid and more watery so allowing sperm through. The cervix also becomes more open.

Sperm production is a continuous process and it only takes one to two days from each ejaculation for the 'count' (numbers of sperm) to be back to its original level. If sperm are not ejaculated they age, becoming less healthy, and eventually die. The less often a man has sex, the higher the proportion of aged and unhealthy sperm in his semen.

The journey to the egg

The journey to the egg is a long and dangerous one, which is why the *motility* (mobility) of the sperm and their health are as important as their numbers.

At least 95 per cent of the sperm either leak out of the vagina or are killed by its secretions. A million or so make it through the cervix to the womb where most of them will be killed by white blood cells (the cells that kill germs). Only a hundred or so will make it to a fallopian tube.

Sperm can reach the tubes in under five minutes but aren't ready to fertilize an egg until several hours after ejaculation. This is because they have to go through a process called *capacitation* in which they lose the skin covering their head and the movements of their tail become stronger.

They can survive in the woman's body for up to four days, or even longer, and this gives some leeway in the timing of sex since the egg is only fertilizable for a few hours, 24 at most.

Fertilization

To be ready for fertilization the egg must be fully mature and at the right place – in the top half of the 4 inch (10cm) fallopian tube – where it has been wafted by fine hairs called *cilia*.

The sperm move towards it and one manages to get through its tough outer layer. This causes a chemical reaction which stops any other sperm doing the same.

The egg draws the sperm further in and over the next few hours the sperm and egg fuse with each other.

The early days of the embryo

Glossary

oocyte	immature ovum
gamete	sex cell – sperm or ovum
ovum	singular of 'ova'
zygote	newly fertilized ovum
morula	fertilized ovum that is a ball of identical cells
blastocyst	fertilized ovum that has gone beyond the morula stage and prepares for implantation; its outer layer of cells attach to the womb and the inner layer go to make up the baby
pre-embryo	the embryo before implantation
embryo	general term for the baby in the first two months of pregnancy (strictly speaking after implantation)
foetus	the baby from two months after conception until birth

Over the next few days this cell or *embryo* divides many times while moving down the fallopian tube, so that after four to five days when it enters the womb it is made up of about 32 cells. It has not yet grown in size however.

Up until the time when the embryo has more than eight cells, each of these cells could produce a complete, identical person. Identical twins are produced if the embryo splits into two, identical triplets if it splits into three, and so on. Non-identical twins are made if two eggs are released and fertilized at the same time.

The pregnancy can be detected at this very early stage in a blood test (and later in a urine test) because the embryo starts producing the hormone *human chorionic gonadotrophin* (*HCG*). This hormone keeps the empty follicle pumping out progesterone. Oestrogen levels also keep on rising.

Figure 5 shows hormone levels after conception.

Implantation

Seven to eight days after fertilization the embryo starts to *implant* itself in the womb lining, which is ready thickened to feed it. About 40 per cent of pregnancies are lost at this point and if you have a period that is slightly late or heavier than usual this may be what has happened.

By 14 days the embryo is firmly embedded in the womb lining, which keeps on building up under the influence of progesterone. As the pregnancy goes on miscarriage (loss of pregnancy) becomes less and less likely.

The developing embryo

Now the embryo starts to develop. Only some of its cells go to make up the baby. Others make up the *placenta*, the disc of tissue which forms on the womb lining, and the *umbilical cord* which connects the baby to the placenta.

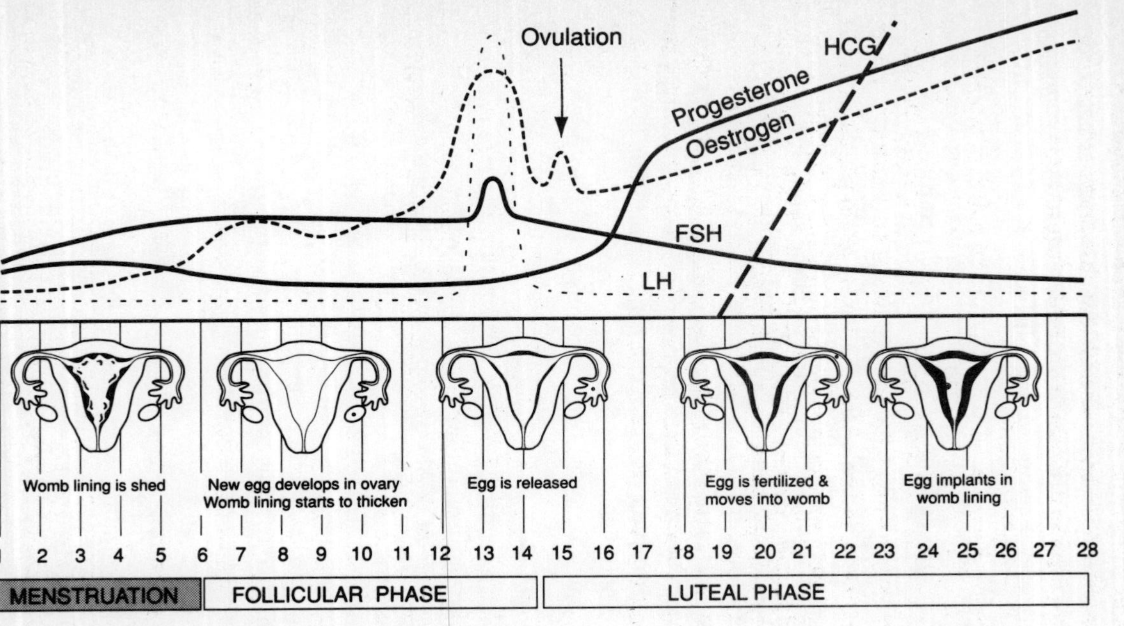

Fig. 5 The menstrual cycle with pregnancy

The first signs of organs forming in the embryo are called the 'primitive streak' and this stage is often considered the one at which life really begins.

From embryo to foetus

By two months after fertilization the baby, now called a *foetus*, is no longer directly connected to the womb lining. It feeds and discharges waste through the placenta. This is to protect its own delicate circulatory system from the pressure of the mother's and to provide a filter for some (but not all) of the harmful substances that might come its way. The empty egg follicle stops sending out progesterone and finally dies.

This is conception when all goes well, but it doesn't always do so and the next chapter describes some of the things that can go wrong.

CHAPTER 3

What can go wrong

The causes and symptoms of infertility in men and women

There are many reasons for infertility and couples may have a combination of problems.

The main causes

According to a 1992 report by Bristol University in the UK the main causes of infertility are:

- sperm defects/dysfunction (24 per cent)
- ovulation failure (21 per cent)
- damage to the fallopian tubes (14 per cent)
- endometriosis (6 per cent)
- problems with cervical mucus (3 per cent)

Infertility in women

Ovulation failure

Ovulation failure or *anovulation* is one of the biggest causes of infertility in women, accounting for about a third of cases. The main symptoms are:

- lack of periods (*amenorrhoea*)
- infrequent periods (at intervals of more than 36 days) (*oligomenorrhoea*)
- frequent periods (every 24 days or less)
- very light periods (with hardly any bleeding)

Frequent periods are not necessarily a sign that anything is wrong. It is possible but uncommon to have apparently normal periods but not be ovulating – to have 'anovulatory cycles', in medical terms.

The main causes of ovulation failure are:

- malfunction of any of the glands connected with reproduction – the hypothalamus, the pituitary or the ovaries
- malfunction of the adrenal glands or, occasionally, the thyroid gland
- tumours or cysts in any of the glands.

Polycystic ovary syndrome (PCOS)

This is the biggest cause of ovulation failure.

A fifth of women have many cysts ('poly' means many) on their ovaries without them causing problems, but in PCOS the cysts are part of a vicious circle of hormone imbalance.

The syndrome may be inherited and being overweight can bring it on. Women with PCOS tend to have irregular periods or none.

Because PCOS causes the ovaries to produce extra male hormones (they produce some anyway) sufferers may have acne and more face and body hair than normal. They may also have a tendency to put on weight.

High prolactin

Prolactin is a hormone produced by the pituitary to stimulate milk production in pregnancy. Some non-pregnant women have high levels and this can stop their periods. High levels can be caused by drugs such as heroin, tranquillizers and indigestion remedies as well as malfunctioning glands.

The contraceptive pill

Two per cent of women have permanent ovulation failure when they come off the pill. This is more likely if you started taking it young (in your teens) before your periods were properly established, had erratic periods anyway beforehand, or took it erratically – stopped and started it several times.

Health and wellbeing

Too much exercise over a length of time can stop periods as can being over- or underweight. *Bulimia nervosa*, even if your weight is normal, can also upset them. Bulimia can also cause PCOS. (Bulimia is binge eating with self-induced vomiting or overuse of laxatives.)

Mental strain can stop ovulation – for instance a third of women having fertility tests and treatment have an increase in the number of anovulatory cycles.

Damaged fallopian tubes

Tubal damage accounts for about a quarter of female infertility in the UK and nearly half in the US. In the US it is the biggest single cause of infertility in women. Tubal damage can result from:

- pelvic inflammatory disease
- pelvic and abdominal surgery
- abdominal disease, eg appendicitis, peritonitis, colitis
- ectopic pregnancy
- endometriosis (see page 25)
- sterilization

Pelvic inflammatory disease (PID)

This is an umbrella term for any infection of the reproductive organs and is the most common cause of tubal damage. *Salpingitis* is a specific term for tubal infection. PID is thought to be caused by:

- sexually transmitted diseases
- infection after miscarriage, abortion or giving birth
- infection from the insertion or removal of a 'coil' or *intra-uterine device* (IUD)

- infection from micro-organisms naturally found in the body.

The faster you get proper treatment for PID the less likely it is to damage tubes. Symptoms are a temperature, pelvic pain and unusual bleeding or vaginal discharge. Unfortunately most women with PID do not have acute symptoms and some do not have any symptoms at all. Some women have chronic symptoms such as low backache, painful periods, pain on love-making, tiredness and cystitis-like pain when urinating.

Sexually transmitted diseases (STDs)

STDs damage the reproductive tubing in both men and women and can affect the baby in the womb. STDs cover a wide range of infections from genital warts and pubic lice ('crabs') to the much more serious gonorrhea and syphilis. The most common STD, though, is *chlamydia*, an infection named after the group of micro-organisms that cause it.

As many as 70 per cent of women and 50 per cent of men with chlamydia have no symptoms and the disease can lie dormant for many years. Symptoms if you do get them include a discharge from the vagina or penis and pain on urinating.

If you think you might have come in contact with an STD – even if it was a long time ago – the quickest and easiest way to be checked out is to go to the genito-urinary (GU) clinic of your local hospital.

Most can be treated with antibiotics (and obviously your partner needs to be treated as well).

Ectopic pregnancy

This is where the embryo starts to develop outside the womb, usually in one of the tubes. It can itself be caused by a damaged tube which stops the embryo moving into the womb. It can also happen if you become pregnant with a coil in place.

An ectopic pregnancy is very dangerous and causes severe pain. It must be surgically removed as quickly as possible, preferably before the tube bursts as this can damage the other tube as well.

If the tube is not too badly damaged it may be left in but this increases the risk of another ectopic pregnancy.

Problems with other reproductive organs

The cervix

Cervical mucus problems – sometimes called 'hostile mucus' – include the following:

- The mucus does not thin properly at ovulation to allow sperm through.
- It contains antibodies that the woman has produced to her partner's sperm which kill the sperm.
- Cervical infections kill sperm or make the mucus too acidic for them.

If the cervix is damaged or weak it can allow infection into the womb and cause miscarriage. This is called having an 'incompetent cervix'. You can be born with a weak cervix. Miscarriage and childbirth can damage the cervix.

The womb

Fibroids – non-cancerous tumours in the womb – are common in older women and needn't necessarily cause any problems. Doctors are not sure why they cause infertility but it may be because they distort the shape of the womb or block the opening to the tubes. They can cause heavy and painful periods or swelling in the abdomen.

Some women are born with an abnormally shaped womb. This is more likely to cause miscarriage than a failure to conceive.

A quarter of women have a *retroverted* womb (one that is tilted backwards). This does not cause problems.

Endometriosis

This is when the womb lining (*endometrium*) starts growing in other parts of the abdomen where it creates scarring which distorts the reproductive organs and stops them working properly.

It is the cause of a fifth of female infertility and is mostly likely in women aged between 30 and 40 who have not had children. It may be inherited. It leads to painful periods and painful sex.

Miscarriage

One in five pregnancies ends in miscarriage, three-quarters of these happening in the first twelve weeks.

After one miscarriage you are statistically no more likely to miscarry again than the average but with each miscarriage after that the chances of it happening again are greater. The risk also increases with age.

Doctors call miscarriages 'abortions'.

All bleeding in pregnancy should be investigated but it is very common and needn't mean miscarriage.

Doctors don't really know why miscarriages happen but suspect:

- an abnormal egg or sperm
- a damaged ('incompetent') cervix
- an abnormally shaped womb
- hormone deficiencies
- immune problems (the woman's body rejects the baby as 'foreign')
- drugs, alcohol, radiation, chemicals, smoking
- illness and stress

Premature menopause

This is when the ovaries stop working or the woman runs out of eggs. It can happen at any age. The woman's periods stop completely and she may have menopausal symptoms like hot flushes and a dry vagina.

Premature menopause can be caused by serious damage to the ovaries from infection, radiation or cancer drugs. Or it may be that you were born with fewer eggs than normal or have a tendency to discard more each month.

Another cause, not properly understood, is *autoimmunity* when the body attacks its own cells. This may be behind as many as half the cases.

Infertility in men

Sperm quality and quantity

Sperm disorders are the biggest single cause of infertility and the problems doctors are least able to treat. They account for nearly three-quarters of male infertility.

Because sperm counts have dropped so dramatically since the 1960s, doctors have revised normal fertility downwards. Normal fertility is now 20 million sperm (per millilitre of semen) and above. Having too few sperm is called *oligospermia*.

Quality and quantity of sperm tend to go together – a man with a low sperm count is more likely to have poor quality sperm. (But remember, sperm quantity does not necessarily relate to the quantity of semen produced.) Sperm quality is measured in terms of ability to move (*motility*) and shape (*morphology*).

Motility is important because sperm must move quickly through the hostile environment of the vagina and be able to penetrate the cervical mucus. Morphology is important because abnormally shaped sperm may not be able to fertilize the egg or if they do may cause miscarriage or birth defects.

The reasons for sperm disorders are not properly understood but doctors suggest:

- age, health and environment
- varicocele
- infection
- autoimmunity
- hormonal problems
- congenital conditions

Age, health and environment

As a man ages he produces more abnormal sperm. Heat, illness, being overweight, drugs, excessive exercise and stress can all cause a reduction in the numbers of sperm produced. Pollution may also play a part.

Varicocele

This is a collection of swollen veins, like a varicose vein, above a testicle, usually the left-hand one. Sometimes it is big enough to be felt or seen and sometimes not.

Ten per cent of all men, whether fertile or infertile, have varicoceles but 30 to 40 per cent of men with fertility problems have them.

It is thought they damage sperm production by causing the testicle to overheat.

Infection

This is suspected when there are extra white blood cells (part of the body's defence system) in the semen but often the actual organisms cannot be identified. Microbes of the *mycoplasma* type may be particularly harmful.

Autoimmunity

This is when the man's body attacks his own sperm, causing them to cluster or 'clump' together. This is known as sperm *agglutination*. It causes up to 30 per cent of male infertility.

Hormonal problems
These are less common in men than women (10–15 per cent of infertile men).

Congenital conditions
The number of sperm-generating cells is fixed when a baby boy is in the womb so any damage at that stage can have repercussions on his sperm output in adulthood.

Sperm transport

Tubal blockage
This is the cause of ten per cent of male infertility. The blockage can be a birth defect or from injury but is usually the result of disease, especially sexually transmitted types (see box on page 23). There may be no sperm in the semen or too few.

Retrograde ejaculation
This is when semen is ejaculated backwards into the bladder. It is not common (one per cent of male infertility) but sometimes happens as a result of surgery to the prostate or urethra, nerve damage, diabetes or drugs, particularly tranquillizers or those to control high blood pressure.

No sperm

Complete lack of of sperm – *azoospermia* – is rare, happening in under five per cent of men. It is caused by:

- a malfunctioning pituitary gland
- injury to the testicles
- mumps during or after puberty
- undescended testicles
- birth defect of the testicles

Injury to the testicles can cause permanent sterility unless quickly treated. Only five per cent of men who get mumps are actually left permanently sterile. Undescended testicles need to be operated on when the boy is very young. Even so there may be something wrong with them which stopped them descending in the first place.

Unexplained infertility

The infertility of up to a third of all couples seeking medical help is diagnosed as 'unexplained'. This means one of three things:

- There is no problem and the couple have just been unlucky so far.
- There is a problem but the tests have not managed to pick it up.
- The problem is one that doctors don't yet know about.

All this is very complicated, but there are many simple things we can do for ourselves both to improve natural fertility and to cure some of the most intractable problems, as the next chapter explains.

CHAPTER 4

How to help yourself

Making the most of natural fertility

This chapter covers the three areas where you can make a difference:

- lovemaking – when and how
- a healthy lifestyle – going one step further
- natural therapies you can do at home

Lovemaking

A normally fertile couple is able to have sex as and when they feel like it and still have a reasonable chance of conceiving. Unfortunately, a subfertile couple must be a bit more calculating – and this in itself can cause problems.

Counselling, psychotherapy and hypnotherapy can all help sexual problems, whether minor or severe. They are covered in Chapter 8.

When

As explained in Chapter 2, women are only fertile when they ovulate. This usually happens 14 days before the start of the next period, whatever the length of the cycle. Unfortunately few periods arrive on the dot so it is difficult to know exactly when the time of ovulation is likely to be.

Although sperm can probably survive in the woman's body for as long as four days, an egg only stays viable for 12 to 24 hours after ovulation. So how can we tell the best time to have sex?

In the past this was a fiddly business involving the woman taking her temperature every morning. And the trouble with this technique is that it is retrospective – that is, it tells you that you have ovulated after you have done so.

Now on the market, however, are 'ovulation prediction tests' which measure the pre-ovulation LH surge in your urine. Although these are expensive, they can tell you are likely to ovulate in 24 to 36 hours' time. If you then have sex at any time during the next two to three days you will maximize your chances of pregnancy.

Unfortunately it is not easy to spot a positive result in isolation so keep all your completed tests and date them so that you can compare one with the other. You may also want to show them to a doctor.

Another new device is the 'Baby Comp' which is a combined thermometer and mini-computer. It tells you when you are most fertile.

Doctors consider a 'regular cycle' to be one that is 26 to 34 days long and does not vary by more than four days from one cycle to the next (although in one survey almost two-thirds of the women had cycles that varied by more than eight days). If you have a regular cycle you will almost certainly be ovulating. If you have very irregular cycles you may still detect the LH surge but you will probably not be ovulating.

A simpler but less precise way for women to tell the fertile period is through their cervical mucus. This may start to feel damp a few days before ovulation. At first it will be white or yellow, then cloudy and finally clear. The clear, wet mucus coincides with peak fertility.

Some women notice other changes in their bodies around the time of ovulation. These include:

- lower abdominal pain
- increased *libido* (sexual feelings)
- 'spotting' (slight discharges of blood, as in a period)
- breast tenderness

A 'natural family planning' teacher can help women recognize the signs of fertility in themselves (see appendix B).

If you find this all too much, the simple advice is to have sex every other day, bearing in mind that the most fertile period is around the middle of the cycle – that is, between nine and 15 days after the start of the woman's last period in a 28-day cycle.

Every two days is the best spacing of intercourse – for two reasons:

- sperm take about two days from ejaculation to regain their previous levels and so if a man has sex every day the counts are reduced
- any longer and the proportion of older, less effective sperm in the semen is greater

One hint for women suffering from endometriosis is to time sex slightly earlier than normal – about day 8 – as the sperm have a more tortuous journey to make in a body damaged by the disease.

How

Doctors disagree as to how many of the following technical refinements really make a difference and obviously they are only worth worrying about during the fertile period.

- The man shouldn't have a hot bath immediately before sex as this will depress the sperm.
- Don't use lubricants as these can kill sperm.
- The best position for bringing the sperm into contact with the cervix, unless the woman has a retroverted

uterus, is for the woman to be on her back with a cushion under her behind. If she has a retroverted uterus it is better for the man to enter from behind.

- If the woman has an orgasm while the man is ejaculating or afterwards this will help to draw the sperm into the cervix.
- The penis should stay in the vagina until it is flaccid (limp) so as not to pull any semen out too soon.
- The woman should not douche the vagina (wash with a water jet, as in a bidet), or urinate, immediately after intercourse.
- The woman should stay lying down afterwards for at least half an hour and preferably longer.

Men suffering from retrograde ejaculation could try having sex with a full bladder.

A healthy lifestyle

Simple leaflets on getting fit for pregnancy are readily available from doctors and chemists. Good health in both the man and the woman will not only give your baby the best start in life but will also give you a better chance of conceiving.

Foresight, the charity concerned with pre-conception care and natural methods of combating infertility, has more detailed advice including:

- eating a very healthy diet
- taking food supplements where necessary
- avoiding pollution
- cutting out drugs (alcohol, cigarettes, some medication, street drugs)
- being tested for genito-urinary infection as this may be behind some sperm problems and cervical mucus problems

Diet

A healthy diet is low in fat, particularly animal fat, sugar and salt, refined carbohydrates and processed foods. Simply, this means doing the following.

- Cutting down on meat and dairy products like cheese and milk and substituting them with fish or vegetable protein (nuts, pulses, grains).
- Cooking with oils such as olive or sunflower rather than butter or lard.
- Eating wholemeal bread and pasta and brown rice, rather than the white alternatives.
- Having as much fruit and vegetables as possible, as fresh as possible and preferably raw.

Most of these products are now available from supermarkets and there are many vegetarian cookbooks available which will explain all the different ingredients, including one from Foresight.

Processed food is not only depleted of its nutrients but contains many additives that are harmful – one look at the ingredients lists should be enough to put you off. It also tends to have lots of salt and sugar in it.

Ready-cooked meals, tinned food, most shop-bought cakes, biscuits and desserts, crisps and other savoury snacks, spreads, fizzy drinks, ketchups, sauces and mayonnaise are all 'processed food'. If lack of time is your problem, there are healthier, vegetarian ready-made items in wholefood shops.

To keep fruit and vegetables fresh, store them in the fridge (except for root vegetables which can be stored unwrapped in a cool, dark place). Frozen produce may be better than unfrozen that is several days' old.

Honey or concentrated fruit juice (available from wholefood shops) can be used instead of sugar. Beware of added sugar in supposedly healthy things such as fruit juice and breakfast cereals.

Oil should be 'cold pressed' and margarine should be '*non*-hydrogenated'. This is to preserve the types of fat essential to our health called 'essential fatty acids' (EFAs).

Weight

If either the man or the woman is over- or underweight, this can affect their fertility.

In men, being too heavy is worse than being too thin as excess fat can cause testicles to overheat and so upset sperm production.

In women being overweight can actually stop periods. If you are too thin, according to Margaret Leroy in the UK magazine *What Doctors Don't Tell You*, 'you may not be menstruating, you may be menstruating but not ovulating, you may be menstruating and ovulating but will have difficulty conceiving, or you may manage to conceive but will have difficulty carrying a pregnancy to term'.

Figure 6 shows the ideal weight range for both men and women. (Where you fall in the range depends on the size of your frame.) A healthy diet should, over time, regularize any weight problems – but don't expect instant cures. If your problem is severe you may like to get help from your doctor, a natural health practitioner or an eating disorders association.

As already mentioned, erratic eating such as in bulimia can also damage fertility.

Avoiding pollution

Radiation

Both men and women should have the minimum of x-rays as these can lead to an increased risk of miscarriage. Men should avoid x-rays to their pelvic area at all times as this can disrupt sperm production. Women should only have x-rays in the first half of their monthly cycle in case they are pregnant without knowing.

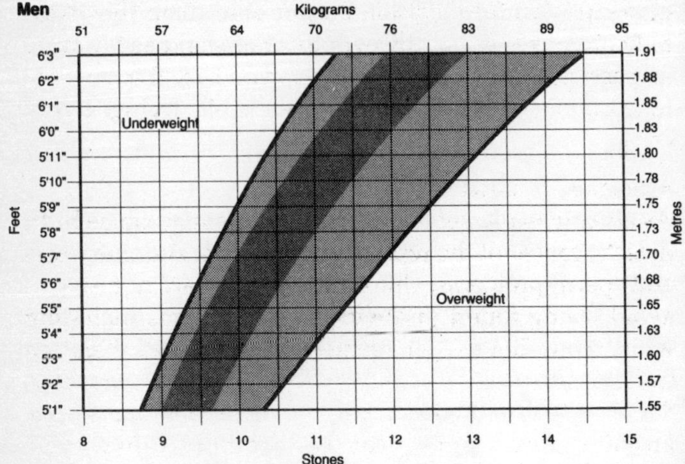

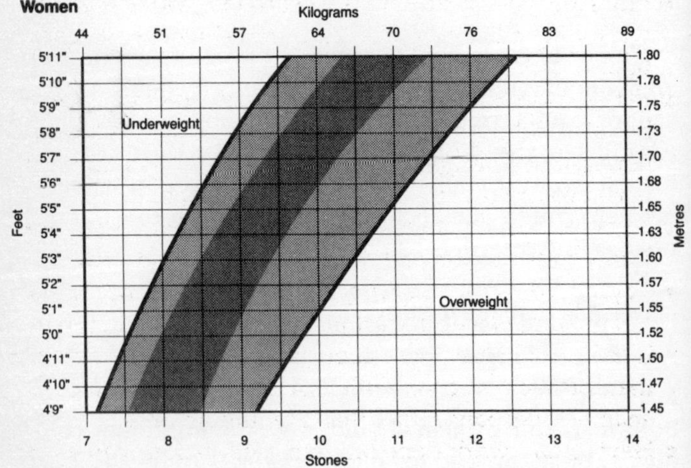

Fig. 6 The ideal weight ranges for women and men

Computer screens, microwaves and televisions also give out harmful radiation but are safer than they used to be. It makes sense however to sit or stand as far away as possible from the appliances as you can. It is best not to use sunbeds and electric blankets while trying to conceive.

Metals and chemicals

As already explained, oestrogen mimics may cause birth defects, cancer of the reproductive organs, endometriosis and sperm problems. Unfortunately they are not easy to avoid, being found in a wide range of items including white tooth fillings, detergents, pesticides (and therefore in food) and plastic packaging as well as drinking water. Some metals, particularly lead and cadmium, have been linked in studies with fertility problems of all kinds.

Ways to avoid pollution include the following.

- Filtering your drinking and cooking water – either with a jug filter or with a filter fitted to your kitchen tap.
- Eating 'organic' produce, not just fruit and vegetables, but also pulses, seeds, bread, dairy produce and meat. 'Organic' or 'organically grown' means something has been produced without pesticides or drugs.
- Avoiding smoky atmospheres, places where there are lots of traffic fumes and driving too much yourself.
- Trying to avoid buying too much food or drink wrapped in plastic, in cartons lined with aluminium or in tins. At home, store food in china or glass rather than plastic and cook with cast iron, stainless steel or enamel saucepans rather than aluminium ones.
- Having any work done on your teeth before you start trying for a baby or, if this is not possible, women should have it done in the first half of their cycle. This applies to both mercury and white fillings.

Nutrient	Good Food Sources	Comments
Vitamin A	eggs, butter, yellow and dark green fruit and vegetables	Deficiency causes damage to sperm-producing cells or ovaries. Too much can be toxic.
B vitamins	wholegrains, seeds, nuts, pulses, yeast, some vegetables, mushrooms	Depleted by contraceptive pill. Very important for hormone system, especially pituitary gland. B12 good for combating low sperm counts. Don't take supplements of just one B vitamin (take a B complex) – they work together.
Vitamin C	raw fruit and vegetables	Fights infection, stress, pollution and ageing. Particularly good for combating sperm abnormalities, agglutination and poor motility.
Vitamin E	cold-pressed oils, wholegrains, green leafy vegetables	Improves sperm function and ovulation.
Essential fatty acids	evening primrose oil (supplement), cold-pressed oils (eg olive oil), oily fish, avocados, sunflower and sesame seeds	Help reduced sperm motility and low sperm counts and may help endometriosis. Work best with suplements of vitamins B6 and C, magnesium and zinc.
Iron	eggs, fish, dried fruit, dark green leafy vegetables	Low levels associated with infertility in women.
Manganese	wholegrains, nuts, onions, parsley	Depleted by contraceptive pill. Important for implantation of embryo.
Magnesium	milk, nuts, seafood, wholegrains	Depleted by contraceptive pill. Helps B vitamins to be absorbed.
Selenium	herring, tuna, wholewheat, broccoli, garlic	Strengthens immune system and fights inflammation. Try for endometriosis, hostile mucus, sperm problems. Take with vitamins A, C and E to help absorption. Harmful if you take too much.
Zinc	seafood, milk, wholegrains, dried fruit	Essential for sperm production and motility. Low levels in women cause implantation failure and miscarriage. A deficiency may contribute to the eating disorder, anorexia nervosa.

Fig. 7 Some of the nutrients connected with fertility

Taking supplements

All pollution increases our need for nutrients, particularly vitamins and minerals. Figure 7 shows some of the nutrients connected with fertility.

Sometimes eating healthily is not enough and we need to take supplements. Research studies have shown that remarkable improvements in fertility can result from large doses of vitamins and minerals. However, self-prescription can be very confusing and some of the nutrients (vitamin A and selenium for example) are dangerous if you take too much. Chapter 7 goes into nutritional therapy in more detail.

Foresight will do an analysis of your hair to see which nutrients you are low in and whether you have high levels of metals. They will then draw up a programme of supplements for you.

Drugs

Alcohol can affect male and female fertility and contribute to miscarriage. It is particularly bad for sperm. Ideally both of you should cut it out completely or have no more than one or two drinks a week.

Smoking harms the fertility of both men and women and is a major cause of abnormal pregnancies.

Marijuana interferes with sperm production and the effects take three to nine months to wear off. Other street drugs are probably best avoided as well – by both men and women – as many can damage chromosomes and so cause birth defects or miscarriage.

Caffeine has a mixed press. One study at Harvard University in America showed that women who drank two cups of coffee a day decreased the chances of conceiving a baby by half. However they all eventually became pregnant and another study showed no link at all between coffee and fertility. Coffee does, however, deplete our bodies of minerals and in pregnancy women are advised to keep their consumption down. Caffeine is also found (in smaller amounts) in tea, cola drinks, chocolate and some painkillers.

Some *prescribed drugs* can stop sperm production and ovulation or reduce sex drive. Check with your doctor.

Heather and Nick's story

My first pregnancy progressed without any problems and I gave birth to a beautiful 8lb 14oz (4kg) boy. However both my next pregnancies ended at thirteen weeks and I was enormously upset. The doctor in charge of my case said, 'Oh, but we have women in here who have six or seven miscarriages'. Quite how this was supposed to help was beyond me.

Then a friend told me about Foresight and after hearing my story they said the problem was probably lack of zinc. This just stunned me. No one at the hospital had suggested anything could be done.

The results of the hair analysis were that I was desperately low in zinc and that Nick was slightly low. In my case it was probably the result of three things – the pill, drinking too much coffee and the miscarriages themselves. We were prescribed zinc supplements for three months, and advised to use a barrier method of contraception, eat a very healthy diet, filter our water, take more exercise and drink no alcohol.

I would say that our diet had always been pretty good anyway but now we paid enormous attention to eating healthily. It wasn't an ordeal at all. All Foresight emphasizes is the importance of whole, unadulterated and unprocessed foods, organically produced where possible. Lots of starches and lots of fresh fruit and vegetables. Nick wasn't too keen on stopping alcohol, however, and we did have a few drinks over Christmas. I started swimming two or three evenings each week.

We both felt really healthy and my periods which had always been pretty erratic suddenly became totally regular – 28 days on the dot.

At the end of the three months I conceived very quickly and after a lovely pregnancy produced our second son who weighed in at 10lb 14½ oz (4.95kg). Three years later, after more preconception care from Foresight, our daughter was born, weighing in at a mere 10lb 4oz (4.65kg).

I told my dad about Foresight a little cautiously as he is definitely not a lentil and sandals man. He keeps a flock of sheep and when I mentioned the zinc supplements he said, 'But that's what we give to the sheep'. Apparently if there are instances of spontaneous abortion farmers give them a 'mineral lick'.

Of course I might have had a successful pregnancy without the Foresight programme. I will never know. What delighted me was that both Nick and I could do something positive to improve our chances.

Foresight has been attacked as an organization of middle-class parents trying to produce 'super babies'. I take great exception to this. People who have stillborn babies or miscarriages are often just desperate for a healthy baby. Most of us would do anything to achieve that. I wish that this sort of advice was available to everyone as part of a pre-conceptional care programme.

Natural therapies you can do at home

Below are some simple suggestions for keeping yourself up to par mentally and physically at this difficult time.

Exercise

The best therapy of all is regular exercise – preferably at least two or three times a week. This doesn't have to be strenuous, but do try to get out of breath as this is good for the heart and lungs. Try walking or swimming as these are relaxing at the same time.

As mentioned before too much exercise can stop ovulation and sperm production – moderation is the key (as in most things).

Breathing

If you find yourself getting tense and worried do some deep slow breathing, through the nose rather than the mouth, and into the stomach not the chest. Or you could try the following simple yoga breathing exercise.

1 Breathe in slowly and deeply through the nose while counting up to four in your head.
2 Hold your breath for a count of four.
3 Breathe out slowly through the nose for a count of four.
4 Wait for a count of four.
5 Repeat as many times as you like.

Concentrating on the counting and the pattern will calm your mind, while the regular breathing will calm your body. (For more about yoga see Chapter 9.)

Relaxation

If you find it difficult to relax, treat yourself to a relaxation cassette – these are available in many shops and through mail order (look at the advertisements in health magazines).

Self-hypnosis tapes can be even more effective although make sure you get a reputable one, preferably through a therapist, as hypnosis is a powerful tool. Some are specifically for fertility. (See appendix C.)

Massage and aromatherapy

Massage – either of self or partner – is very therapeutic and often recommended for sexual problems. You can learn it from a book or just do what feels good. If you combine it with aromatherapy it is even nicer. (For more about massage and aromatherapy see Chapter 7.)

For massage, aromatherapy oils need to be diluted. Put approximately two drops of 'essential' (scented) oil with ¼ pint (5ml) or ½ cup of 'base' massage oil. Grapeseed oil is ideal for the purpose and readily available. You can use a few drops of neat essential oil in the bath.

To be on the safe side, you should avoid the oils which must not be used in pregnancy. These are basil, clove, cinnamon, fennel, hyssop, juniper, marjoram, myrrh, pennyroyal, peppermint, rosemary, sage and thyme.

Those safe in pregnancy and good for fertility are:

- citrus oils (bergamot, grapefruit, lemon, neroli, orange) – refreshing
- chamomile – soothing for the skin and the mind
- frankincense – an exotic rejuvenating oil, calms the mind
- geranium – good for balancing the hormones and the emotions
- lavender – the cure-all oil, helps fight infection
- rose – cleansing, good for many sexual and menstrual disorders
- sandalwood – encourages self-expression, especially good for men
- ylang ylang – aphrodisiac, gives confidence

Choose the scents that appeal to you and mix them if you like.

Having done all you can by yourself, you may decide to go further. The next chapter covers the tests and treatment offered by conventional medicine.

CHAPTER 5

Conventional medical tests and treatments

What they feel like, how successful they are and what the side effects or dangers are

Although men account for half of fertility problems, the burden of conventional treatment falls on women. The process is very drawn out, taking months if not years, as the tests are done at specific times of the month and in sequence.

Going to your family doctor

This is probably your first port of call. Your doctor will do some simple tests and may prescribe some drugs. Then, when the doctor (or you) thinks it necessary, he or she will refer you to a specialist.

Physical examination
In the woman the doctor will be feeling for cysts, fibroids or damage to any pelvic organs. In the man he or she will be looking for any malformation of the organs, lumps, a varicocele or infection.

Blood test
The woman is tested for her levels of oestrogen, progesterone, LH, FSH, prolactin, testosterone and thyroid hormone. The test is usually done on day 21 (seven days

before the start of your *next* period) and may be done more than once.

Semen analysis

Popularly known as a 'sperm count', a semen analysis involves the man masturbating into a small bottle which then has to be wrapped in cotton wool to keep it warm and taken to a laboratory (usually at the local hospital) for analysis within an hour. He may be asked not to have sex for a day or two beforehand. Sperm counts are very variable so the test may be done more than once.

Figure 8 is an example of a sperm analysis: you will probably have to ask if you want to see a copy of your own results. The result shown has been classified, surprisingly, as 'moderate'.

Normal Values	Results
Volume (1–5ml)	3.8ml
pH (7–8)	7.7
Liquefaction (liquid)	liquid
Count (> 20M/ml)	8.5M/ml
Motility (> 50% motile)	32%
Morphology (< 30% abnormal)	51%

Fig. 8 Example of a semen analysis

Going to a specialist

If you are lucky you will be treated together. However, very often different medical specialisms are involved and the man will go to see a *urologist* and the woman a *gynaecologist*.

Women

Post-coital test (PCT)

This is done around day 14 of the woman's cycle. She may be given oestrogen to stimulate cervical mucus. Six to 12 hours after the couple has had sex a sample of the woman's cervical mucus is taken, in a procedure rather like a cervical smear. (Showering is allowed before the test but not a bath.) This is to show:

- whether the woman is producing mucus of the right sort (liquid enough for the sperm to get through)
- how the sperm react to the mucus – can they move through it; does it kill them?
- whether you're actually having sex properly

Basal body temperature (BBT) recording

The woman is asked to take her temperature first thing every morning and record it on a chart. This is to check ovulation since the temperature rises then.

Ultrasound scan

This is used to view the ovaries and maturing eggs, both as a check on them and as part of certain treatments. Advanced equipment can check the fallopian tubes as well. It is said to be quite safe, having been used for several decades, although it can temporarily disrupt the menstrual cycle.

A probe is either placed on the abdomen or passed up through the vagina. If the former, the woman has to have a full bladder (as water is a good conductor of sound).

Hysterosalpingogram (HSG)

This is used to check the womb and tubes. Radioactive dye is injected through the cervix into the womb and watched by x-ray as it passes into the tubes.

It can be very painful. The radiation can increase the risk of birth defects. The test can spread infection into the very areas you need to keep clear of infection. On the other hand it can actually clear obstructions.

Laparoscopy ('lap')

With the woman under general anaesthetic, a small cut is made in her navel and a viewing tube called a *laparoscope* inserted so that all the pelvic organs can be inspected. At the same time minor surgery can be done or tissue samples extracted for further study.

There is a complication rate of 1.1 per 1000, mainly puncturing of the internal organs and life-threatening bleeding.

Men

Split-ejaculate semen analysis

The initial spurts of semen are richer in sperm than the later so the man has to masturbate into two bottles – not an easy thing to do – so that the first part of his ejaculate can be tested separately (or used for assisted conception).

Testicular biopsy

A piece of tissue is taken from each testicle with the man under general anaesthetic. This is to check sperm production at source rather than in the semen so as to find out whether there is a blockage in any of the tubes.

Vasography

A check for blockages of the two vas deferens using radioactive dye and x-ray, carried out with the man under general anaesthetic. Usually done at the same time as a testicular biopsy.

Blood tests

These are to check levels of FSH, LH, testosterone, prolactin and thyroid hormone.

Drug treatment

(Where brand names are given, the drug name is in brackets.)

Women

Oestrogen

This is given as pills or vaginal creams to stimulate cervical mucus production and make the mucus more watery (and so penetrable by sperm). It doesn't necessarily work and it may disrupt ovulation.

Duphaston, gestone, proluton (progestogen)

These are all synthetic progesterone, given by injection or vaginal pessary (a tablet you insert into the vagina) to women who tend to miscarry or have an 'inadequate luteal phase' (they do not produce enough progesterone after ovulation for the womb lining to build up). Researchers at King's College Hospital in London in 1993 found that they had no effect whatsoever.

They are also given after embryo replacement in assisted conception.

Steroids

These are sometimes given to women to suppress sperm antibodies in their cervical mucus. Steroids have serious side-effects and should only be taken for short periods.

Clomid, serophene (clomiphene)

The first and most famous of the fertility drugs, used to stimulate ovulation and sometimes to counteract progesterone deficiency. They are taken as pills for about five days of each cycle.

Ovulation is induced in 80 to 90 per cent of women but only 30 to 40 per cent become pregnant. This may be because the drugs also cause the cervical mucus to thicken. Oestrogen is sometimes given at the same time to try and counteract this.

The risk of multiple pregnancy (non-identical) is one in 20 (normal risk is one in 80) – mostly twins but occasionally more. A 1988 study by Serono, the company which makes serophene, found there was a 2.5 per cent risk of birth defects compared to the normal average of 1.8.

It can make you feel sick or giddy or have hot flushes. If you have blurring of your vision or bad pelvic pain (caused by the ovaries enlarging – a 14 per cent risk) you must stop taking it immediately. It can make endometriosis and PCOS worse. It triples the risk of ovarian cancer.

Similar drugs are *nolvadex* and *tamofen* (tamoxifen) but these are more expensive so are only prescribed if you react badly to the others. They can cause womb cancer.

Gonadotrophon LH, pregnyl, profasi (human chorionic gonadotrophin – HCG)

Sometimes used with Clomiphene. Used in assisted conception. It is injected and can actually stop ovulation if given at the wrong time (even by a few hours).

Parlodel (bromocriptine)

Used to bring down high prolactin levels. It is taken as pills, can make you feel very sick, but leads to pregnancy in 70 per cent of women with high prolactin.

Humegon, normegon (human menopausal gonadotrophin – HMG); Pergonal (menotrophin)

The 'superovulation' drugs, usually given if other fertility drugs haven't worked and for assisted conception. They are injected every one or two days or administered via a small pump which the woman wears continuously.

The pregnancy rate is 60 per cent, but with a greater risk of miscarriage than normal. There is a 25 per cent risk of multiple pregnancy (five per cent risk of three or more).

Another, serious, risk is *ovarian hyper-stimulation syndrome* (*OHSS*) which can not only permanently damage ovaries but can be fatal. To avoid these you should be monitored with scans several times each cycle and possibly blood (or urine) tests.

The drug increases your risk of a stroke. The risk of ovarian cancer is tripled and there is an increased risk of breast cancer. It is too early to be certain about long-term effects but fears include premature menopause and ovarian cancer. The long-term effects on the child, particularly its reproductive system, are not yet known.

Metrodin, orgafol (urofollitrophin/FSH)
As HMG and menotrophin. May be helpful for PCOS.

Fertiral (LHRH/GNRH)
As HMG and menotrophin but with smaller risks of multiple pregnancy or OHSS. Pump administered only.

Suprecur (buserelin)
Synarel (nafarelin)
These are also called *LHRH/GNRH analogues* and are used to shut down the natural action of the pituitary gland before treatment with the superovulation drugs, either where these haven't worked on their own or before assisted conception. May be helpful for PCOS.

You take them by nasal spray every four hours or so.

Side effects include hot flushes, dry vagina, breast tenderness and headaches.

Danol (danazol)
The drug most often used to treat endometriosis. It is taken as pills.

At least a fifth of women experience side effects. These include menopausal symptoms, excess hair growth, weight gain, greasy skin and irreversible voice deepening.

You can't get pregnant while on the drug and when you stop it the endometriosis tends to return. However, 30 per cent of women with severe endometriosis and 60 per cent with mild endometriosis will conceive after the treatment. (In the case of mild endometriosis this is only slightly higher than the rate of pregnancy without treatment.)

The contraceptive pill, progestogens and LHRH analogues are also used for endometriosis.

Men

Antibiotics

These are sometimes tried for sperm problems as genito-urinary (GU) infections lower sperm counts and cause sperm abnormalities. Foresight lists 16 separate infections for which you and your partner should be tested and treated.

Steroids

These are sometimes prescribed if the man produces antibodies to his own sperm. Although, as mentioned before, they have unpleasant and serious side effects, large doses for short periods of time are fairly successful – the partners of a third of men so treated will become pregnant.

Pro-viron (mesterolone)

A synthetic male hormone often prescribed for low sperm counts but with very little success. It is taken as pills. There is a risk of liver cancer.

Restandol, sustanon, virormone (testosterone)

Taking testosterone reduces sperm production but sometimes there is a 'rebound effect' after treatment with half of men having a temporary improvement in sperm count. There is a slight risk that sperm production will be permanently stopped. Restandol comes as pills; the others are injected.

Pergonal (menotrophin)
Humegon, normegon (HMG)
Gonadotrophon LH, pregnyl, profasi (HCG)
Orgafol (FSH)
Parlodel (bromocriptine)
If you have a hormone deficiency, these can be fairly effective – a third of men will have improvements in sperm count, but possibly not sperm motility.

Clomiphene and tamoxifen
Sometimes prescribed for low sperm counts but they are not very successful. They can cause permanent sterility.

Other treatments

Women

PCOS
There are two surgical treatments for PCOS if drugs don't work. The first involves cutting a wedge out of the ovaries and the second burning off the cysts. With surgery through a laparoscope or microscope (microsurgery), both are now fairly successful (70 per cent chance of pregnancy).

Blocked fallopian tubes
With microsurgery, there is a 25–50 per cent chance of correction depending on the type of damage. However not all types of damage are suitable for surgery and after surgery the risk of ectopic pregnancy is increased.

Sterilization
Surgery to reverse sterilization is 65 to 95 per cent successful if the tubes were cut, tied or clipped. If they were sealed with heat however the chances of success are less.

Tim and Julia's story

We got married in our early twenties (reports Tim) and although I didn't particularly want children we never used any contraception. Julia wanted children very much as her parents had both died when she was a child and she wanted a proper family life. As the years went by we began to wonder if anything was wrong but were reluctant to go the doctor as Julia was overweight and she thought they would just tell her to go away and lose weight before they would treat her.

Eventually we went and had the usual basic tests. We were told Julia was not ovulating and she was put on clomiphene for about 12 months. By this time she was 30 and when nothing happened we were referred to the fertility clinic at the local hospital. There they diagnosed Julia as having polycystic ovary syndrome. We were devastated and furious at all the time we'd lost.

The hospital decided to do a laparoscopy to check Julia's tubes and to burn off some of the cysts with diathermy – this was only a short term solution as the cysts would grow back. Julia was absolutely petrified of having a general anaesthetic and we had to wait a year for them to fit us in.

Following the laparoscopy Julia was put on buserelin and metrodin, one to shut down the natural action of the pituitary and the other to mature the eggs. Luckily I'm a nurse so I could give her the metrodin injections but she still had to go to the hospital for scans all the time and carry the buserelin spray around with her.

We had to make love to schedule – when the eggs were ripe – which was terrible. At one time I actually thought I was paralysed because I couldn't do anything! I was working nights at the time so not only was I feeling dreadful – I'm always like a bear with a sore head – but it was extremely difficult to make sure we were together at the right time.

We're still having active treatment and the next step is IUI. We couldn't afford to pay for any more drugs ourselves or for IVF. We've thought about adoption but I feel angry about all the vetting we'd have to go through. Anyway, we'll soon be too old.

We've joined the fertility clinic support group and I have spoken about infertility on television. I think secrecy only makes things worse and the more we can get the media interested the more treatment hospitals are going to offer. It's time the authorities realized that infertility is a health problem just like anything else and just how many people there are out there suffering from it.

Cervical mucus problems

An alternative (but perhaps not very practical one) to steroids is the woman is producing sperm antibodies in her cervical mucus is for her partner to wear a condom for several months, even a year.

If the cervix is infected a new treatment being tried by some doctors is to remove the infected mucus glands by laser and then use drugs to stimulate new non-infected ones to grow.

Fibroids

These can be removed by surgery but the pregnancy rate after treatment over the age of 35 is only 35 per cent (and fibroids do tend to be found in older women). There is a risk of excessive bleeding in the womb afterwards.

Abnormally shaped wombs

A *septate* womb has a protrusion from the top. It can be easily and successfully corrected with minor surgery.

Some women have a double womb. This needs very specialized surgery but if properly performed can be fairly successful.

Endometriosis

Minor endometriosis reduces fertility by half compared with normal and treatment does not really help.

The damage from severe endometriosis can be corrected surgically but may return. Conception rates after laparoscopic laser surgery or microsurgery are 70 per cent.

Miscarriage

An incompetent cervix can be stitched shut early in pregnancy and the stitches removed before the birth. This is usually successful.

Premature menopause

There is no treatment. A few women recover spontaneously.

Men

Sperm problems

Doctors will usually advise you:

- not to have hot baths
- to wear loose fitting underwear and trousers
- to spray your testicles with cold water twice a day

Sometimes this is enough to make a difference.

Varicocele

This can be tied off or blocked, with either general or local anaesthetic. Eighty per cent of men will have an improvement in sperm afterwards but only half will get their partners pregnant. Results are best if your sperm count was moderate beforehand (ie above 10 million per ml) and showed the typical varicocele pattern – immature, dying and dead sperm. The full benefits usually take about six months to show.

Tubal blockage

Surgery is difficult as the tubes are so small but 20 to 30 per cent of men will have raised sperm counts afterwards. However if the tubes have been blocked for a long time the testicle tends gradually to stop producing sperm.

Vasectomy

Male sterilization is a simple operation in which the two vas deferens are blocked. Unblocking them is much more complicated and, although usually successful, pregnancy only follows in about a third of couples. This may be because two-thirds of men have sperm agglutination afterwards.

Assisted conception

In vitro fertilization (IVF)

This is the original 'test tube baby' technique, first done successfully in 1977.

An egg or (more usually) eggs are removed from the woman by vaginal ultrasound with local anaesthetic or the woman sedated. The eggs are mixed in the laboratory with fresh sperm and left for two to three days. A quantity of fertilized eggs (maximum three in the UK) are then placed in the woman's womb through the vagina and cervix – no anaesthetic is needed for this.

The woman is usually treated with superovulation drugs beforehand to stimulate extra eggs to mature and HCG to 'prime' them and then with progestogen or HCG for two weeks afterwards to 'support' the pregnancy.

The technique was developed for women with blocked tubes. It is now also used for endometriosis, cervical mucus problems, sperm disorders and unexplained infertility.

It is very expensive and not covered by health insurance in many countries – though in Britain it is sometimes available on the National Health Service. The chances of a live birth per treatment are 10–15 per cent, less if the woman is over 40 or the man has sperm problems. More than one embryo is replaced to increase the chances of success but multiple pregnancies run a greater risk of miscarriage, premature birth and low birth weight babies.

Too many embryos are usually produced and the couple has four choices about what to have done with them. They can be:

- frozen for their own future use (not very successful)
- donated to another couple
- donated for research (in some countries only and, in the UK, only up until they are 14 days old)
- destroyed

Gamete intra fallopian transfer (GIFT)

This is similar to IVF but the eggs are collected from the ovary by laparoscope with the woman under general anaesthetic and then immediately placed in the tubes together with some sperm. It is simpler (and therefore cheaper) to do but the woman must have healthy tubes. Success rates may be slightly higher than for IVF.

Zygote intra fallopian transfer (ZIFT)

A combination of IVF and GIFT – embryos, or zygotes, are placed in the tubes. It is more complicated to do than either IVF or GIFT and success rates are no higher but it may be helpful for older women.

Intra uterine insemination (IUI)

A sample of fresh semen is placed in the woman's womb through the vagina without anaesthetic. It is used for cervical mucus problems, mild endometriosis, slightly below average sperm and unexplained infertility.

The woman usually goes through the superovulation process beforehand as this gives better results but as fertilization takes place naturally has to be very carefully monitored in case too many eggs are produced (in which case the treatment is abandoned for that cycle).

Live birth rates are 10 per cent.

Micro assisted fertilization (MAF)

These are the newest treatments, used for severe male sperm problems. A few or even just one sperm are injected into an egg. If there is a tubal blockage in the male, sperm can even be taken from the epididymis for use. (This is known as *micro epididymal sperm aspiration* (MESA).) The woman goes through the normal superovulation and egg retrieval procedure.

The most successful MAF technique so far is *intra cytoplasmic sperm injection* (*ICSI*), followed by *sub zonal insemination* (*SUZI*), with *partial zonal dissection* (*PZD*) the least successful.

There are concerns that the techniques are escalating before they have been properly tested. Researchers at a Dutch university in 1995 found that the foetuses of five out of 12 women who conceived through MAF were showing abnormalities, several of these due to the sperm – which may have been the cause of the fathers' infertility in the first place.

Sperm and egg donation

Sperm donation

Donated sperm are usually introduced into either the woman's cervix or her womb (IUI), either with superovulation beforehand or without.

Egg donation

Egg donation is more difficult because the woman donating her eggs has to go through the same superovulation and surgical procedures as in IVF. In the UK she is not allowed to be paid for this and so there is a shortage of donated eggs.

The recipient is prepared for pregnancy with hormones; the eggs are fertilized in the laboratory and then introduced transvaginally as in IVF. The technique can be used for post-menopausal women.

The law on sperm and egg donation varies from country to country and is being changed all the time.

Having described the conventional medical answers to infertility, and given you some idea of what you can do for yourself, the book now turns to the natural therapies with their radically different approach to both diagnosis and treatment.

Carolyn and Bob's story

We started trying for a baby when I was 31 and Bob 32 and went to see our family doctor together a year later who referred us to our local Fertility Clinic for tests. I didn't want to go as for several years I'd avoided going to doctors and had used homoeopaths instead. However I felt time was running out.

At the clinic we had a range of tests which took six months. Our diagnosis was 'unexplained', a source of some comfort but frustration as well. I asked to take clomid for six months and we then had two goes at IUI. That didn't work so we went up to a London teaching hospital for IVF.

We got the treatment cheaply because were part of a research project but I hated the place – it was big, busy and dirty. The drug buserelin gave me hot flushes and my ovaries felt very uncomforatble. We had to stay in London for a week and make several trips for monitoring. The egg retrieval was done with only tranquillizers and painkillers and it was almost unbearable.

The treatment was unsuccessful and I was very ill afterwards with a virus due to exhaustion. I decided to have a course of acupuncture and found a wonderful woman who also prescribed Chinese herbs. She made me feel a lot better both physically and mentally and she was completely sympathetic and supportive towards the IVF treatment.

Three months later we went to a private hospital nearer to home. It cost us three times as much but was worth every penny. I felt much happier about the treatment because I knew what to expect. I asked for much lower doses of the drugs (I'd produced 41 eggs first time round) and had the egg retrieval done under general anaesthetic. Three embryos were replaced, I had a twin pregnancy for twelve weeks, then one healthy baby.

I then had a completely normal pregnancy and, although our daughter was born five weeks early (because my waters broke which is common under any circumstances), she is now a healthy happy baby.

When she was eight months old, quite by accident I became pregnant again and could hardly believe it. It was a completely natural conception and I was in shock for weeks; life can be very ironic. Two babies in two years!

Looking back now I still feel emotional about what happened and feel the pain of the three years I spent wanting a baby and not being able to conceive. It was very traumatic for me accepting 'hi-tech' treatment with powerful drugs and it was a long journey to be able to come to terms with this and embrace it wholeheartedly.

I could not have done it without access to complementary therapies at the same time, which I feel preserve my sanity and my faith in myself. I needed a lot of support and, although my first pregnancy was certainly due to the skill and dedication of the IVF clinic, it was definitely holistic therapies which got me through.

CHAPTER 6

The natural therapies and infertility

Introducing the gentle alternatives

Why go to a natural therapist?

The number of people visiting natural therapists is rocketing throughout the world. In Britain, for example, a recent survey by the Consumers' Association found that one in four of its members had visited a practitioner of natural medicine – nearly double the number who said they had tried natural therapy in a similar survey three years earlier.

Surveys of patients using natural practitioners have found there are two main reasons for turning to these forms of therapy.

The top reason is disappointing experiences with conventional doctors. A Dutch study found that 39 per cent of people using a natural therapist had been unhappy with the service they had received from conventional doctors. The next most common reason was that a friend or relative had recommended the therapy. Some people turn to natural medicine as a last resort.

Interestingly, only a small proportion of patients cited a firm belief in natural therapy as their reasons for going to a natural therapist.

Whatever their reasons for turning to natural therapy,

most people seem to be very satisfied with the treatment they receive. In the UK, the Consumers' Association found that four out of five of its members who used a natural therapist claim to have been cured or to have had their symptoms improved by a natural therapist – and three-quarters of them said they would visit a natural therapist again.

What is natural therapy?

On the surface it sometimes seems that the natural therapies have little in common. For example, what has herbalism – using plants to heal – in common with reflexology – a system of healing through foot manipulation? In fact, although the various therapies use a wide range of techniques, they are all based on a similar approach, as follows.

- Symptoms are assessed in relation to the personality of the patient. The therapist will want to get an overall picture of the patient so that treatment can be tailored to that individual. Unlike conventional medicine, the treatment administered by a natural therapist for a particular condition will vary from person to person.
- The whole person is treated, not just the symptoms. The natural practitioner breaks down the barriers between mind and body and heals the person as a whole. This means he or she will need to make a full assessment of your character, stresses, state of mind and natural energy.
- Many natural therapies are based on the idea that illness happens when the body's systems are out of balance and in a state of 'dis-ease'. The therapy aims to restore that balance.
- Natural therapists are not simply concerned with removing the immediate symptoms but will work to

restore people to a state of health and wellbeing where they will be able to avoid further illness. They recognize that someone who is in poor general health will need more than a quick-fix cure. Often a natural therapist will work with an individual long after the original symptoms have cleared up to help them achieve a higher state of physical and mental wellbeing.

- The goal of natural therapy is self-healing. Most of the therapies recognize that each individual has some power for self-healing that may need to be harnessed more effectively. This also means that patients are encouraged to help themselves. If you are used to visiting a conventional doctor who simply writes out a prescription you may find that a natural therapist will expect more input from you. There is more of a partnership between patient and therapist towards the goal of maintaining good health.

Conventional doctors and the natural therapies

Doctors are becoming more willing than they were to accept that natural therapies have something to offer. The British Medical Association reported in 1994 that nearly three-quarters of British family doctors had referred a patient to a natural therapist at some time and that 80 per cent of trainee doctors wanted to train in one or more of the natural therapies in addition to their conventional training.

Estimates of the number of doctors actually practising natural therapies range from 2 to 15 per cent. In the UK the number of medically qualified doctors who also practise homeopathy has risen from 200 to more than 1,000 in less than a decade. Although that is a very small proportion of the 35,000 family doctors in the UK, the numbers are still rising.

However, even though more doctors are taking up the practice of natural therapies, most people will still have to seek out a specialist in the various natural therapies rather than a doctor for treatment.

What to expect when you see a natural therapist

The most striking difference between natural therapy and conventional medicine is the length of time you will spend in consultation with your therapist. A first consultation with a natural therapist is likely to take at least an hour and much of that time will be spent finding out about you and your life. Further consultations are unlikely to be as long as the first but will still be longer than you would spend with a doctor.

Treatments are different too. Often, after the initial problem has cleared up, you will continue to receive some form of therapy aimed at restoring your body's natural healing ability. For this reason treatments may take longer than those used in conventional medicine – although in the case of infertility where tests and treatment can be drawn out for months, if not years, this may not be so.

In addition to specific treatments you will usually be advised to make changes to your lifestyle – for example, a change of diet or sleeping habits, stress management and exercise may all be recommended to help you back to good health.

You will not be a passive recipient of healthcare. You may determine the direction of the treatment since you know more about your own body and mind than anyone and you will be encouraged to take responsibility for your own health.

On the whole the treatments are pleasant in themselves and most are without harmful side effects. You may initially find your symptoms are worse. This is known as a healing crisis and is a good sign because it means your body's defence systems are getting to work.

Do the natural therapies work?

This is one of the most hotly debated issues in medical circles. Natural practitioners are convinced of the benefits of their therapies but they have had a hard time convincing conventional doctors.

Though there are plenty of satisfied customers and practitioners have many case histories to demonstrate the benefits of their work there is little proof in the form of strictly conducted clinical trials.

A clinical trial usually compares a medicine with a dummy pill in patients who do not know which pill they are taking. A dummy pill (known as a 'placebo') which is identical in appearance to the active drug is used because it is known that patients can show an improvement in their condition if they think they are receiving a cure. This is known as the 'placebo effect'. If the medicine is shown to be statistically more effective than the placebo then it can be said to work.

The problem with the natural therapies is that they are often not suited to the strict controls of clinical trials. Firstly the emotional support of the practitioner is seen as an integral part of the treatment rather than something that is muddying the scientific results. Secondly, since practitioners treat different people differently, it is virtually impossible to compare like with like. Finally, it is difficult in some of the therapies to have a placebo group. In acupuncture, for example, how do you give a 'dummy' needle?

Choosing a natural therapy

In some ways it doesn't really matter which therapy you choose. Just to be attracted intuitively to a particular therapy may mean it is the right one for you. Or you may have more conscious reasons for your choice. For example, you may prefer reflexology to an all-over body treatment if you are nervous about being touched by a stranger.

Choose a treatment you will enjoy and then you will be able to relax and cooperate fully with your therapist. This is the very best basis for success.

If you are going to mix the therapies, try and choose ones that are as different as possible otherwise you may be wasting or confusing the effects. Acupuncture and Chinese herbs, for example, are a traditional combination whereas acupuncture and craniosacral therapy, both of which work on the so-called 'subtle energies', could cause more harm than good by either counteracting each other or, more likely, over-stimulating the system. Equally, a physical therapy such as aromatherapy massage would combine beautifully with a mental one like counselling, whereas too many mental therapies would exhaust you.

Therapies for infertility

The following chapters describe the natural therapies that may be helpful for infertility. They have been chosen for three main reasons, because:

- clinical trials show they are effective
- practitioners have used them successfully
- patients have been helped by them

Other therapies have been included because they are among the better known natural therapies and so you are likely to come across them.

However, there are many new natural therapies being developed all the time and even if there is no evidence so far that a therapy helps infertility this does not mean it will not help you. The main disadvantage with the newer therapies is that regulation is less developed so it is more difficult to find a reliable practitioner.

The therapies have been grouped into three to help you understand what they are like, but there is in fact considerable overlap between the groups and all work on different levels at the same time.

Physical therapies

- aromatherapy
- herbal medicine
- homeopathy
- massage
- naturopathy
- nutritional therapy
- osteopathy

Emotional and mental therapies

- flower remedies
- counselling and psychotherapy
- hypnotherapy
- meditation

'Energy' therapies

- acupuncture
- craniosacral therapy
- healing
- reflexology
- shiatsu
- yoga

We start off by looking at the physical therapies.

CHAPTER 7

Treating your body

Physical therapies for infertility

The physical therapies are among the best known natural therapies and those most accepted by the medical profession. In the US, for instance, all osteopaths are also trained doctors and in the UK aromatherapy and massage are being used increasingly in hospitals. Many scientific trials also now are revealing the importance of nutrition to fertility.

Aromatherapy

Aromatherapy uses the 'essential oils' of plants for healing. These oils are what gives plants their fragrance and they can be extracted from leaves, twigs, fruit or flowers, by pressing or by steaming and distillation. They evaporate easily so have to be kept in tightly closed dark glass bottles. Some, such as rose and frankincense, are very precious and are usually sold diluted in a carrier oil. Oils from organically grown plants are best as there is no risk they will have traces of pesticides in them.

The oils are used in cosmetics and therapeutically in massage. They can also be taken internally but this is less usual because of the dangers of doing so with some oils.

Aromatherapy massage is believed to work both on

the body because the oils are absorbed through the skin and on the mind and emotions because of the scents which affect the nervous system. Some therapists consider that the life force of the plant is in the oil and that this energy too can have an effect. For this reason, natural plant oils should always be used, not synthetic versions.

Your therapist will choose a mixture of oils he or she considers suitable for you but don't be shy to say yourself which ones appeal to you. Some of them smell quite peculiar in the bottle but change once on the skin.

Many nurses are now being trained to give aromatherapy massage to hospital patients because it has proved so effective in the treatment of pain, stress and mental disorders. The oils can also strengthen the immune system and balance bodily functions.

The International Journal of Aromatherapy, for instance, reported in 1995 on a woman with PCOS due to have her only remaining ovary removed because of a 5 inch (12.8 cm) cyst who claimed that aromatherapy massage brought it down to ¾ inch (18mm) in two weeks – and that after three to four months it was completely gone.

The journal also reported on a woman with endometriosis who was free of continual pain and able to lead a normal life after six months of treatment.

Herbal medicine

Herbal medicine, whether Western or Oriental, has been used for thousands of years and is probably the oldest form of medicine known. In many under-developed countries it remains the main form of medicine. In China it is, with acupuncture, the official mainstream form of medicine.

Many drugs come from herbs but herbs are considered safer for several reasons.

- Our bodies are better able to cope with natural substances than manmade ones because that is the way they have evolved.
- Unlike a single drug, a plant contains many different but complementary active ingredients which can offset any toxic effects.

That is not to say however that herbs are totally without danger – some are very strong indeed – and they should always be taken under expert guidance, especially when pregnancy is a possibility.

The diagnosis

A Western herbalist may make a physical examination or take blood or urine samples. A practitioner of Chinese herbal medicine will take your pulse – in six places on each wrist – and look at your tongue. Both should ask for your medical history in detail.

The treatment

Western herbs will usually be taken as pills or liquids. Oriental herbs are taken as teas – usually very strong and bitter tasting. You have to boil up the herbs to make the teas and this can be quite complicated and time consuming. (Some Oriental 'herbal' remedies are actually from animals – for example, a herbal soup prepared from salted fish heads is prescribed for fevers – so if this worries you be sure to mention it to your practitioner so that he or she can use alternatives.)

Who can it help?

Many herbs act like hormones (eg wild yam) or balance hormone output in the body (eg *Vitex agnus castus*). They can provide a general tonic (eg ginseng for men), boosting the reproductive organs (eg squaw vine for the womb) and increasing sex drive. Some herbalists claim that treatment can even unblock fallopian tubes.

Studies of Oriental herbal treatment reported in various journals including the *American Journal of Chinese Medicine* and the *International Journal of Fertility and Menopausal Studies* show it being effective for: low sperm counts, low sperm motility, semen abnormality, ovulation problems, fibroids, endometriosis, PCOS, pituitary/ovary problems, high prolactin, infertility caused by auto-immunity and unspecified infertility.

Homeopathy

A system of healthcare founded by a German doctor, Samuel Hahnemann, two hundred years ago, this is one of the more established natural therapies with large numbers of doctors practising it in France and Germany. In Britain a growing number of doctors are trained in homeopathy and several hospitals offer it alongside conventional medicine, where it is free under the state health service.

Homeopathy is based on the principle of 'like cures like', a bit like vaccination. The sick person is prescribed minute doses of substances that would produce in a healthy person effects similar to those occurring in the disease. This is said to stimulate the body's own healing powers.

For example, the homeopathic way of treating insomnia is to give a minute dose of a substance such as coffee which in large doses causes sleeplessness.

However, your individual characteristics and symptoms are as important as the label attached to your ailment. Two different people with the same apparent problem are unlikely to be given the same remedy.

There are some 3,000 remedies, made from ground-down plants, minerals, metals and other substances. This powder is diluted with water and alcohol many times and with each dilution the mixture is shaken vigorously

Juliet's story

We started trying for a baby when I was 35. I had no trouble getting pregnant but four months into the pregnancy I had a terrible feeling of doom. When I then started bleeding I knew I'd lost the baby.

My second and third pregnancies both ended at three months. Although all my pregnancies and miscarriages felt completely different, both these times I knew instinctively I wasn't pregnant any more. This was confirmed in the second pregnancy when I started bleeding and in the third one when a scan showed the baby had got smaller – it had actually died in the womb.

In the third pregnancy they took the baby out before I'd started bleeding and throughout the nine months when I would have been pregnant I had terrible pains like labour pains whenever I should have been having a period. Once I had to be rushed to hospital by ambulance.

It was during this time that I went to see a homeopath. It was wonderful to find somebody who treated me holistically and I feel it was as a result of his treatment that I finally had a normal period – strangely enough around the time that the baby would have been due. I was very relieved as I had thought my fertility was gone for good.

For the fourth pregnancy my doctor referred me to a specialist who gave me extra progesterone at six weeks. I continued seeing the homeopath and at nine months, when I was 40, my son was born.

I can't say whether it was the homeopathy or the extra progesterone that got me through my fourth pregnancy but I do know that the homeopathic treatment was a tremendous psychological support.

> My son is now four years old and I'd love to have another baby but feel it would be risky at my age and wouldn't want to put my husband through any more stress. I take part in a miscarriage helpline as I want other women to know that there are ways to avoid these terrible tragedies. I'm just thankful I made it in the end.

– 'succussed'. The more the mixture is succussed the more powerful it is said to become.

No trace of the original substance can actually be detected in the final mixture but homeopaths believe that it has left an imprint of its energy in the liquid and this is enough to cure. The liquid is usually then soaked into tablets.

These tablets are tasteless and are dissolved on the tongue. While receiving homeopathic treatment you will probably be asked not to take any drugs or eat or drink strong-tasting things like coffee, chilli and peppermint (including in toothpaste) as these can interfere with the action of the remedy.

The remedies are completely harmless and non-addictive. You may however notice an initial worsening of your symptoms or even a recurrence of past symptoms. This is all to the good and a sign that the remedy is working.

There have been scientific studies of homeopathy and infertility and it has been shown to be helpful for:

- hormone problems
- sperm disorders (low sperm, abnormal sperm, sperm with poor motility)
- endometriosis
- fibroids

Practitioners report its effectiveness for:

- low sperm numbers and sperm agglutination
- miscarriage
- sexual problems, physical and mental, in men and women, including painful intercourse
- abnormal periods (eg heavy, painful, infrequent, light)
- cervical mucus problems
- pelvic and genito-urinary infection
- scarring and distortion from past infection
- malfunctioning reproductive organs or glands
- infertility after a debilitating illness
- unexplained infertility

Massage

This is one of the oldest forms of healing and also, today, one of the most popular natural therapies. Not only has it been shown to improve circulation, relax muscles, aid digestion and speed up the elimination of waste products but it also makes us feel better emotionally.

It helps aromatherapy oils to be absorbed and the vapours to be released. In addition, there is a school of thought that says we store painful emotions from the past in our bodies, tensing unnecessarily without realizing, and that massage can free this.

The standard Western form is Swedish massage so called after the Swede, Per Henrik Ling, who developed the techniques last century. There are also many types of Oriental massage, based on Eastern ideas of energy flow in the body. Some of these are described in Chapter 9.

Most massage is entirely painless although you may feel a little uncomfortable when sore spots are touched. There are more violent forms of massage such as 'rolfing' which can be painful.

You need only take off as many clothes as you feel comfortable with – perhaps having just a neck and shoulder massage for your first session.

Naturopathy

Naturopaths are the 'general doctors' of natural medicine. Naturopathy is based on the ideas of 19th-century European doctors who revived ancient Greek principles of good health based on the importance of clean water and air, good food, exercise and relaxation.

Pure naturopathy, or 'nature cure', involves treatments that include fasting, special cleansing diets and hydrotherapy (treatment with water – for example hot or cold baths, compresses, body wraps or inhalation). But most modern naturopaths – the term was coined by European practitioners who went to America at the beginning of the 20th century – also use a wide range of therapies such as osteopathy, homeopathy, herbalism, nutritional therapy (see below) and acupuncture (see Chapter 9).

Many use alternative forms of diagnosis such as iridology (examining the irises of the eyes) or applied kinesiology (muscle testing).

Apart from Britain, where the idea is proving slow to catch on, 'naturopath' is now the term used for a practitioner specializing in natural medicine in its widest sense in the same way 'family doctor' describes a general practitioner of conventional medicine.

In countries such as America, Australia, New Zealand, South Africa, Israel and Germany, naturopaths usually follow a full three- to four-year training along similar lines to conventional doctors.

Nutritional therapy

This therapy uses general dietary improvement, special diets, nutritional supplements and herbs to cure ill-health.

Why do we need it?

- Allergies can stop us absorbing food properly.
- Pollution can increase our need for nutrients.
- Processed food is depleted of nutrients.
- Unless it is organically grown, food can be lacking in essential minerals.
- The 'recommended daily allowances' of vitamins and minerals are probably too low for life in the modern world. We all have different needs and our needs vary greatly at different times of our lives and depending on the amount of stress we are under.

How does it work?

Special diets are used for short periods to 'cleanse' the body and detect allergies. For example:

- fasting
- eating nothing but raw fruit and vegetables
- excluding foods known to cause allergic problems like wheat, yeast and dairy produce and then reintroducing them gradually

Megadoses of vitamins, minerals and other nutrients make good deficiencies and help us break out of the vicious circle of poor health and poor food absorption. These can usually be discontinued or cut right down once health is restored.

Who can it help?

An increasing amount of research is showing the importance of nutrition to sperm production. For example in a 1995 study at the University of Sheffield in the UK men on a three-month course of vitamin E had a significant improvement in sperm function.

US nutrition expert Dr Mervyn Werbach, writing in the *International Journal of Alternative and Complementary Medicine* in 1995, reported that the following research results indicated the value of nutrition in problems of infertility even further.

- Fifty-seven per cent of men whose sperm count was below 20 million responded to daily injections of vitamin B12.
- 1000mg daily of vitamin C increased sperm counts and motility and helped correct sperm agglutination abnormalities and immaturity.
- Out of 14 men who received four months of zinc supplements all had improved sperm counts and the wives of two conceived.

A 1991 UK government survey found that British women of childbearing age were particularly deficient in the nutrients associated with fertility: B vitamins, vitamin E, iron, magnesium and zinc. In the same year researchers from Portsmouth Polytechnic in England reported that low blood iron levels in women are associated with fertility problems. Seven women having trouble getting pregnant conceived after being given iron and vitamin C to treat hair loss.

Again in Britain, a survey by Surrey University on the work of Foresight, the charity concerned with preconceptual care and infertility, found that 81 per cent of couples with previous histories of miscarriage or infertility who had been trying for a baby for up to ten years went on to give birth to healthy babies after following a Foresight diet and supplement programme.

Foresight recommends their programme for:

- sperm and ovulation problems
- unexplained infertility

- those going in for assisted conception
- women with a history of miscarriage
- older couples

Dian Mills, who has done research into endometriosis and nutrition, reported in the newsletter of the UK National Endometriosis Society in 1994 that women who took supplements showed a 98 per cent improvement in symptoms. Supplements need to be geared to the individual, she said, but B vitamins, vitamins C and E, calcium, magnesium, selenium and zinc seemed to help most.

Catherine, with PCOS, went on a six-month course of organic wholefoods and supplements through Foresight, then conceived after her second cycle of clomid. She now has a healthy daughter. Catherine says,

> I firmly believe that the six months of excellent diet and balanced supplementation contributed very significantly to the successful outcome of my treatment.

Alice, who found she had blocked tubes after a miscarriage, decided not to bother with an operation because her husband was against it and because she was told it had only a 30 per cent success rate. She went on a strict Foresight regime of healthy eating and supplements and started going to a gym twice a week. Within six months of being told she would never have children she conceived and later gave birth to a healthy boy.

The UK magazine *Here's Health* reported in 1995 on a woman with hostile cervical mucus who, told she would be unlikely to conceive, became pregnant after twelve months of nutritional therapy.

The difference between dieticians and nutritional therapists

Dieticians work with doctors. Their advice is not geared to the individual but to a particular complaint – for example heart disease. The advice is general and aimed at preventing conditions rather than curing them. They do not diagnose problems themselves.

Nutritional therapists work with individuals, giving detailed advice which takes into account the whole profile of a person's health, not just the main symptom. They aim to bring about long-term improvement.

Osteopathy

This uses massage and 'manipulation' to correct muscles, ligaments and sinews that have become tense or joints that have moved out of position. This can happen through injury or general wear and tear or because of emotional tension. Manipulation means pushing, pulling and twisting different parts of the body. It is gentle and generally quite painless.

Osteopathy can help fertility by increasing blood flow to the organs connected with reproduction and by releasing 'adhesions' – scar tissue caused by infection which can distort the shape and so upset the functioning of organs. It can also realign a badly positioned womb and correct hormone problems.

A derivative is *cranial osteopathy*, which is concerned mainly with the bones of the skull. Another, craniosacral therapy, is covered more fully in Chapter 9.

Osteopathy was developed by a Dr Andrew Taylor Still in America in the last century as a reaction against the harmful medical practices of the time. In America it is now the second largest single natural therapy practised, after chiropractic, with all US osteopaths being trained doctors as well. In Britain it became the first natural therapy to be regulated by law (in 1993), putting osteopaths nearly on a par with doctors and dentists.

Osteopathy compared with chiropractic and physiotherapy/physical therapy

Chiropractors deal with the musculo-skeletal system like osteopaths but with more emphasis on the spine and nervous system. Their manipulation is more forceful and they don't use massage. They are also more likely than osteopaths to use x-rays in their diagnosis. Gentler versions, popular in Britain, are McTimoney chiropractic and McTimoney-Corley chiropractic. There is no evidence of any form of chiropractic helping fertility.

Physiotherapists (as they are called in the UK) or *physical therapists* (in the US) work with doctors and may use machine equipment in their treatment. There is no evidence physiotherapy/physical therapy can help correct infertility.

Having looked at the therapies that approach health through the body, we now turn to the therapies that work primarily on the mind and emotions.

CHAPTER 8

Treating your mind and emotions

Psychological therapies for infertility

Before doctors knew as much as they do now about infertility, and when infertility was considered mostly a woman's problem, doctors thought that nearly half was caused by emotional problems. That view is now unfashionable. Natural therapists, on the other hand, do not separate mind and body and some even believe that *all* health problems stem from the mind and so can be cured by the mind.

Science is discovering the complex interactions between mind and body. It is known that psychological stress causes the release of hormones such as adrenalin and cortisol which suppress our immune defences making us more susceptible to disease. When we tense our muscles we restrict blood flow to parts of the body and stop organs working properly.

Emotional problems may be holding us back without us realizing it. If we are not clear about why and if we want a child we may refrain from sex just at the fertile time without being aware of what we are doing. One counsellor and hypnotherapist treating a woman who kept having miscarriages discovered that she did not trust her husband to be a father to her children because he was violent. The therapist suggests there is a connection.

Of the therapies covered in this chapter, counselling, psychotherapy, hypnotherapy and meditation are all now well established with known effectiveness. The many flower remedies – of which the Bach remedies are the original and the best known – are popular and though unproven in medical trials, have benefit according to the many people who use them.

Counselling and psychotherapy

Counselling is simply a formal way of having someone to talk to but often it is more effective than just talking to a friend. A trained counsellor is able to listen in a more detached, unbiased and honest way than someone who is involved in your life. In addition you have the reassurance that whatever you say is in complete confidence and will not be repeated.

Counsellors can be trained in specific areas such as partnership difficulties, sexual problems, or problems with parents or children. In Britain assisted conception clinics provide counsellors to help couples explore treatment options and their ethical problems, such as what to do with spare embryos or what to tell a child who is the result of sperm or egg donation.

In most countries psychotherapists are really counsellors by another name although they tend to treat more long-standing problems – and in America at least they tend to have a higher status than counsellors, slightly below that of psychologists. They are not to be confused with *psychiatrists* who are medical doctors and treat mental disorders with drugs or surgery (as well as charge considerably more for their services!).

Counsellors and psychotherapists will not tell you what to do but by asking the appropriate questions will help you to discover your own mind. They may also teach you new techniques for coping with life so that you don't keep on repeating the same old behaviour and making the same mistakes. The aim of the therapy is to make you more in control of your life and happiness.

There are many different types of counselling and psychotherapy but probably the most important criterion is whether you think you will get on with the person and be able to trust them. Try and meet them before you decide to go ahead – many therapists offer free initial consultations. Your family doctor may be able to recommend someone.

As with all the natural therapies, you do not have to have a 'problem' to take advantage of counselling or psychotherapy. They can help you to see things in a new way and provide support at any time.

Flower remedies

The original remedies – and still the best known – were developed by a British doctor, Dr Edward Bach (pronounced 'batch' – not as for the composer), in the last years of his life between 1930 and 1936. The 38 different 'Bach flower remedies' he produced are intended to cover all the negative states of mind that people feel.

There are now more than 100 flower remedies produced under the names of about two dozen producers in some 50 countries, but all are based on the same principles of treating first and foremost psychological states as those established by Bach.

The remedies are made from infusions of wild flowers but so diluted as to be completely safe. They are intended for self-prescription.

You take the remedies with water at least four times a day. You can mix different ones together but probably not more than six. When choosing a remedy it is important to take your personality into account, not just your passing moods, so that you can heal your 'whole self'.

The remedies are widely available in most natural health stores in their relevant countries. Further information is available from the Flower Essence Society in California, USA, which maintains a world-wide database of flower remedies, or the Bach Centre based at Dr Bach's former home in Oxfordshire, central England (see appendix B).

Judy Howard, who works at the Bach Centre, includes detailed suggestions on remedies for infertility (for men and women) in her book *Bach Flower Remedies for Women*. The following are some examples:

- *Impatiens* for frustration
- *Gentian* for disappointment
- *Elm* to restore faith and confidence
- *Agrimony* to soothe inner turmoil, particularly for men who hide their feelings
- *Olive* for fatigue
- *Mimulus* for known fears, such as before treatment

The following remedies are also said to help sexual problems:

- *Centaury* for feeling you do not have a right to have sexual needs
- *Heather* for being over-demanding
- *Water violet* for shyness
- *Crab apple* for feeling the body is unclean or shameful

The Bach 'Rescue Remedy' is a mixture of five remedies to be used in emergencies for comfort and calming. It is either drunk in water like the other remedies or can be rubbed on the skin.

Hypnotherapy

Hypnosis is a form of deep relaxation in which you become more in touch with your own feelings.

Initially you will need the help of a trained therapist to reach the right level of relaxation but a good therapist will encourage you to do the same for yourself at home, perhaps with the help of self-hypnosis tapes.

Once in this relaxed state you or your therapist will be able to 'reprogramme' your thoughts and feelings so that you leave behind addictive behaviour patterns like drug abuse or negative thought patterns such as believing yourself to be a failure.

Hypnotherapy can be helpful for sexual problems and for getting rid of harmful habits like smoking, drinking too much, bulimia, and over- and under-eating.

Sometimes you may need to go even deeper, dredging up forgotten incidents from your childhood, for example, which have influenced you ever since without you being aware of it. Now that you are adult you are able to resolve the confusions the incidents created, or to release the emotions that you weren't allowed to at the time. This is sometimes called *hypnoanalysis*.

Rebirthing is the name of a technique that involves going back even further, to your birth, and resolving any pain that this may have caused.

All this can be very useful for future parents, helping them see more clearly their reasons for wanting a child and stopping them repeating the same mistakes that their parents made in bringing them up.

One of the techniques used in hypnosis is *visualization*. This means imagining things as you would like them to be. For example, British therapist Marilyn Glenville described in 1995 in the UK magazine *Here's Health* how during hypnotherapy she asks 'the man or woman to visualize conception, to relax enough to see the possibility that their body can do it. It helps to switch the focus away from temperature charts and timed sexual intercourse'.

UK hypnotherapist Ursula Markham suggests that the therapy can release infertile couples from what she calls 'the treadmill of depression, stress and anxiety' which is such a barrier in itself to conception.

According to Julia Mosse and Josephine Heaton in *The Fertility and Contraception Book,* hypnotherapy and deep relaxation have restarted ovulation in women who were apparently blocking their own cycles.

Hypnotherapy is being used increasingly by the medical profession for pain relief, for psychosomatic illnesses (physical illnesses that may have a mental cause) like asthma, migraine and skin problems, and to help patients cope with treatment, including infertility treatment.

It is very important to trust your hypnotherapist – if you don't the hypnosis won't work. Many hypnotherapists are also counsellors and you might like to spend a few weeks talking about your feelings and getting to know your therapist before actually being hypnotized. Your doctor may be able to recommend a good therapist to you.

Meditation

Meditation is a means of controlling the mind so as to find inner calm and contentment – the sort of feeling you get when you are totally absorbed in doing something you enjoy. At first you practise it in short regular sessions but the aim is for your mind to work like that all the time.

Unfortunately it is not easy. Indian sages say that it is one of our highest achievements as humans and that like sleep it cannot be taught: it comes by itself in its own time. However, you can speed up the process by taking the right steps to begin with.

Meditation is a completely different state of mind from that of the normal daily bustle so it is important to make the distinction. Going to a class, sitting outside, having a special room or miming drawing a pair of curtains can all help.

Sessions twice a day for about 20 minutes are recommended for beginners, preferably after getting up and before going to bed, and at least two hours after a meal.

It is best to have your spine upright, whether sitting or kneeling, otherwise your mind is more likely to wander or you may fall asleep.

There is a huge variety of different techniques for stilling the mind. You can concentrate on breathing deeply and regularly or relaxing every part of your body in turn, or hold a tranquil image in your mind such as a still lake, or chant, or repeat a word to yourself, or look at something calming like a candle.

Stray thoughts should be allowed to wander in and out of your mind. If you try to stop them you are concentrating on them and not on the calming images. Instead, step back and observe them as something separate from your true self.

Meditation gives you time for yourself and time out from the stress of trying for a baby. You may find that fresh insights and new ideas for coping with problems come to you after a session. Meditation can make you feel calmer and more positive about life in general, so helping you put your need for a child into perspective.

It has also been shown to have physical effects, improving functions of the body such as reducing blood pressure and improving circulation. This is all to the good in an area like fertility which, as we have seen, is so sensitive to ill-health of all kinds.

Autogenic training

This system, developed in Canada, combines meditation with positive suggestions and teaches specific mental exercises to encourage relaxation and creativity. But they need to be taught by a qualified therapist. Studies suggest it can be used to increase sperm count.

These are just some of the therapies that work primarily on the mind. The next chapter covers the increasingly popular 'energy' therapies.

CHAPTER 9

Treating your 'subtle body'

'Energy' therapies for infertility

Most of the therapies in this chapter are based on the Oriental idea that around and through our body flows an invisible energy that nourishes the organs just like blood does. This so-called 'subtle energy' is said to be part of the 'life force' that it is believed runs through everything in the universe. In China this energy or life force is called *qi* (pronounced 'chee'), in Japan *ki* and in India *prana*.

Alien as the whole concept is to many Western minds, some form of energy round the body can be picked up by highly sensitive electromagnetic recorders and Kirlian 'photographs', which record electrical fields, also show coloured patterns of light round living things that may relate to this energy.

In acupuncture the energy pathways are called *meridians* and recent research at Beijing University in China has found that the skin is thinner and the nerves different along these meridians.

Just like blood circulating, the energy flow can become too weak in places or too strong or even blocked. Practitioners say this affects the corresponding parts of the body and is related to mental and emotional states. Anything can affect the energy flow – heredity, environment, state of mind, what we eat and drink, infections, even the seasons.

Though we have natural self-balancing mechanisms sometimes we need extra help. So the aim of the different 'energy' therapies is to restore a balanced flow of energy.

Acupuncture

Acupuncture has been used for 5,000 years in China and is still widely used today. It is part of the system of healing called 'Traditional Chinese Medicine' (TCM) which also includes herbal medicine (see Chapter 7).

Acupuncture works by stimulating the flow of *qi* or drawing it away at 365 special points called *acupoints* located on the meridians. This is done either with needles or by burning herbs.

The World Health Organization calls acupuncture 'a clinical procedure of considerable value' and lists it as appropriate for many genito-urinary and reproductive problems including impotence, infertility, premenstrual syndrome, PID and irregular periods. Practitioners say it can also help cysts and fibroids.

Scientific trials have shown acupuncture to be effective for:

- women's hormone disorders
- infrequent periods and lack of ovulation
- poor semen quality
- abnormal semen

Many people are put off acupuncture by the needles but these are actually very fine and the insertion is quite painless. Usually no more than five or six are used at any one time in any case. Sterilization of the needles is of the utmost importance to a properly trained practitioner and many practitioners today use disposable needles.

The herb-burning is called *moxibustion* after the herb *moxa* (common mugwort) which is used. A cone of the dried herb is placed above the acupuncture point (usually on the end of the inserted needle) and lit so that it smoulders from the tip downwards to produce heat on the body. The herb is removed as soon as the patient feels the heat. An alternative method is a stick of the smouldering herb held a short distance away from the relevant point.

On your first visit a good therapist will spend a long time asking you about your medical history, your habits and likes and dislikes. At the same time he or she will be listening to the timbre of your voice, looking at your skin colour, sensing the odour of your body. They will also look at your tongue and take your pulse in six places on each wrist.

According to traditionalists, to be proficient in acupuncture takes a lot of training and experience, and a practitioner should have at least three years' training. A Western form of acupuncture is now in wide use for pain relief and addiction control but this is considered potentially harmful by traditional acupuncturists because they say it suppresses symptoms which will then appear elsewhere in the body in a more serious form.

Craniosacral therapy

Craniosacral therapy was started at the turn of the century by an American osteopath, Dr William Sutherland, who noticed pulsations in the human body coming from deep in the brain and affecting the *cerebrospinal fluid*, the fluid which cushions the brain and spine.

He called these pulsations *craniosacral motion* ('cranio' meaning 'of the brain' and 'sacral' 'of the *sacrum*' – the base of the spine) and saw it as the 'breath of life'. It is carried from the brain and spine throughout the body by the body's connective tissues, with each cell in the body responding with its own particular rhythm.

Therapists feel for imbalances in the motion either by touching you gently or by passing their hands over your body just above its surface. You can stay fully clothed for this. These imbalances can arise from physical injury or emotional tension, past and present.

In the same way that a counsellor provides a sounding board and enables you to find your own answers to things that are troubling you, a craniosacral therapist aims to reflect back to the body its own tensions and enable it to heal itself.

Research is only just beginning into the therapy, mainly in the US, but practitioners say it is ideal for sensitive and painful conditions, both mental and physical, and is perfectly safe in pregnancy.

Mike Boxhall, chairman of the Craniosacral Therapy Association of the UK, believes that craniosacral therapy is very effective at counteracting stress, putting people back in touch with their own bodies and helping them regain the confidence that conventional treatment can take away.

He has worked on about 40 infertile women over the last five years, most of whom had previously received conventional treatment, including IVF. Half of them went on to become pregnant.

Healing

Healing is another one of those therapies, like herbalism and massage, that probably stretches back to the origins of humanity. It is one of the most researched natural therapies and has been proven effective in relieving pain, curing disease and improving people's state of mind.

The UK National Federation of Spiritual Healers claims that it can be helpful in a wide range of physical and psychological conditions whether trivial or serious.

Although miracle cures do happen in healing, you are likely to need several treatments. Some healers actually touch you and some merely pass their hands around your body. You keep your clothes on but may be asked to remove your shoes.

People receiving healing tend to experience the sensations of being re-energized or relaxed, 'pins and needles', heat or coolness, or pain coming to the surface and dispersing.

Some patients begin to feel better as soon as healing begins or shortly after. Others do not feel any benefit until hours or days later. Occasionally healing may take weeks or months before it has any effect. Often symptoms other than the original complaint will also be cleared up.

Spiritual healers believe that the healing is being initiated by a 'higher power' which passes through them to the patient. It is not necessary for the patient to believe this themselves.

In some countries, including many of the states of America, healing for money is illegal. Mainly for this reason healing is more often known as 'Therapeutic Touch' or just 'TT' in many parts of the US. In other countries, even those like Britain where there are no legal limits on healing, many healers do not charge a fee although a donation may be asked for. Genuine healers do not charge exorbitant fees or promise a cure – so beware of any that do.

Healing (or 'TT') is becoming increasingly known and used by doctors and nurses in hospitals in most Western countries, but particularly in Britain and America. A variation finding a wide following in many countries is *Reiki*.

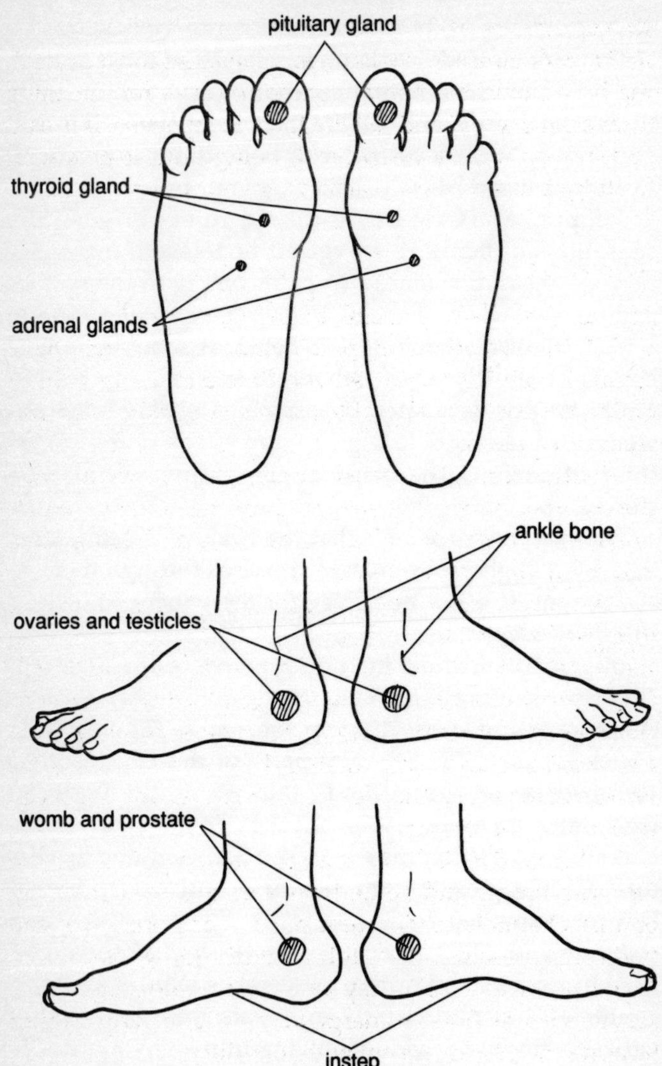

Fig. 9 Reflexology points for infertility

Reiki

Reiki (pronounced 'ray-key') is a Japanese form of healing based on the Oriental concept of qi – 'rei' meaning 'universal energy' and 'ki' life force in Japanese. It is said to work on a very deep level, being both a powerful healing tool and a key to achieving your full potential.

Reflexology

This ancient therapy seems to have a particular affinity with fertility, with many practitioners saying they have found it helpful for all types of conditions including endometriosis, sexual problems, anxiety, and sperm and ovulation problems.

Medical tests have shown that reflexology can produce a wide range of benefits, from improving circulation and digestion to reducing insomnia and depression, and regulating the hormones.

Like acupuncture, it is based on the Oriental idea of energy flow. Earliest traces of the therapy have been found in ancient India, China, Japan, Egypt and North and South America. It was brought to Europe by the Arabs during the Dark and Middle Ages and was then rediscovered and 'relaunched' by the Americans Dr Edward Fitzgerald and Eunice Ingham during the early part of the 20th century.

Reflexologists believe that particular points on the feet and hands and sometimes ears are connected by energy channels to different parts – or zones – of the body. By pressing, massaging and holding the points (usually on the feet) they can release blockages and restore the free flow of energy to the whole body. Figure 9 shows the points helpful with infertility.

The treatment itself is relaxing and non-invasive. You may occasionally feel slight pain on some points which

Holly and Adrian's story

When we'd first got married (reports Holly) I'd had peritonitis but no one at the hospital or our doctor had ever mentioned that it might have affected my fertility. It was my mum who'd eventually come across something in a magazine. By this time we'd been trying for a baby for a year and a half and had been told by the doctor, after basic tests, that everything was normal and just to go away and relax.

It wasn't until a year later that he finally sent us to a specialist who not only confirmed my suspicions about the peritonitis but said that Adrian's sperm counts were not at all good. I was flabbergasted and very upset and felt we'd wasted all that time.

Because of waiting lists it wasn't until ten months later that I had a laparoscopy which showed that my tubes were wrapped in scar tissue and that I also had some endometriosis. I needed treatment but the specialist told me that he had no idea when he could do it as the laser machine was broken and infertility treatment was a very low priority and there was no funding.

I asked if I could have it done privately and two months later had a successful operation.

Adrian had had more sperm counts done and these were much better so we were told to go away and try naturally for a year before we would be considered for further treatment.

I was feeling very stressed by now and when I heard a reflexologist talking at a workshop organized by the hospital's fertility support group I decided to go and see her.

She recommended supplements for us, particularly zinc and magnesium for Adrian and vitamin C for both of us. Every time I saw her I came away so much better – I would be buzzing and feeling I could climb mountains. This would last for a couple of days.

After four weekly treatments we arranged that I would come monthly just before I was due to ovulate so that she could stimulate my ovaries. I used to get sensations in my pelvic area when she did this.

We then went away on holiday and when we got back I had my reflexology treatment and that month we conceived. Telling the reflexologist our news was the best bit about that time as she had taken such a personal interest and was very pleased.

I feel that it was both the conventional and the natural treatment that helped me conceive. I definitely needed to have my tubes seen to but at the same time I needed help on the emotional side – which I certainly didn't get from conventional medicine.

I am astonished that my peritonitis wasn't picked up earlier as a possible problem and think that the doctor knew very little about fertility – you just have to read up all about it for yourself and become your own expert.

It was all very well people telling me to relax but I couldn't until I felt I'd done everything that needed to be done – and that took four years. It was only then that things fell into place.

shows that there is a problem in the corresponding area of the body. You may also have mental reactions such as crying or feelings of calmness.

After the treatment it is quite common to experience sweating, diarrhoea and increased urination for a few days. This is a sign that your body's elimination systems have been stimulated and are flushing out accumulated poisons and waste products. You may temporarily feel lethargic, nauseous or tearful. Again, this is simply part of the healing process.

Shiatsu

Originating in Japan, shiatsu or shiatzu is probably the best-known variation of a type of therapy known as 'acupressure' ('shiatsu' means 'finger pressure' in Japanese). Acupressure, as the name implies, is really acupuncture without needles and has been used for thousands of years, probably longer even than acupuncture. Self-treatment for mild problems is possible. A variation is 'acumassage' which uses massage techniques rather than just pressure.

Shiatsu is a more vigorous form of treatment than acupressure, using the thumbs, fingers, elbows and even knees and feet to apply pressure and stretching to the meridians and acupoints. It usually takes place on a padded surface on the floor and you wear loose comfortable clothing. You can't have the treatment if you are taking steroids.

There may sometimes be pain – showing that there is an energy 'blockage' – and you may have a temporary 'healing reaction' afterwards as toxins and negative emotions are released.

Shiatsu is said to affect all levels of our being so can be used to treat any form of fertility problem, whether physical or mental. As with all complementary therapies, advice on diet and lifestyle is part of the treatment.

According to Shruti Gordon, a practitioner from south-west England who has written a small guide to shiatsu and reproductory issues for the UK Shiatsu

Society, the inability to conceive a baby can be treated quite successfully with shiatsu.

She suggests that as well as receiving treatment couples should work on balancing the mind-body system themselves in preparation for conception. She lists ten steps for doing this which range from stopping smoking, eating properly, resting and exercising to examining your purpose in bringing another child into the world, giving time to self-development and letting go of suffering and neurosis.

She recommends that natural treatments should always be tried *before* conventional ones because the repercussions of conventional treatment will be felt later in life.

Yoga

Yoga is a system of training for body, mind and spirit which originated in India at least seven thousand years ago and is still being developed today.

Hatha yoga, the type most commonly practised in the West, involves postures to train the body, breath control exercises to still the mind and meditation to get in touch with the spirit.

Yoga is said to coordinate body, mind and spirit, so balancing and stimulating the flow of *prana* (life force). Kirlian photography has shown that after a 15-minute session of yoga a person's energy 'charge' increases whereas it doesn't after a similar session of gymnastics.

According to the international research organization Yoga Biomedical Trust, based in London, there is evidence that yoga helps infertility, including low sperm counts and menstrual problems. It is said to improve the blood flow to all the organs and counteract ageing.

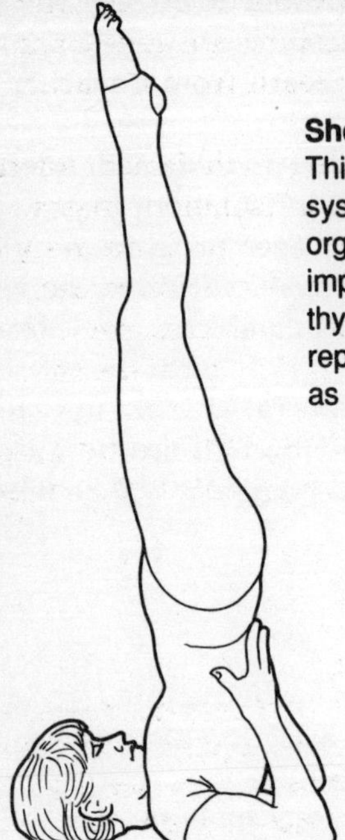

Shoulder stand
This posture rejuvenates the whole system including the sexual organs of men and women. It improves the functioning of the thyroid gland and can help reposition displaced organs such as the womb.

Fish
This tones up the pituitary and the thyroid gland and arrests degeneration of the sexual organs.

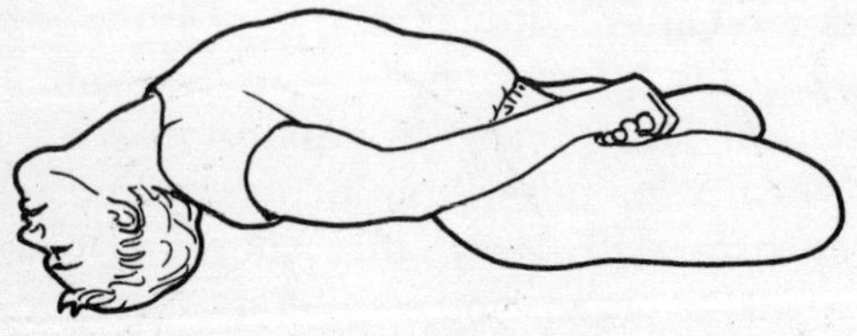

Fig. 10 Some yoga postures for fertility

Yoga can be practised by people of any age and state of health but as some of the postures are quite complicated it is easiest and safest to learn from a teacher in a class.

Figure 10 shows postures that might benefit infertility but it is best not to do them in isolation. Instead you should always carry out a proper programme which includes composing yourself to start with, warming up the body, a balanced selection of postures, some breathing exercises, and relaxation/meditation at the end.

Having decided on a natural therapy, the next step is finding a practitioner you can trust. This is the subject of the next chapter.

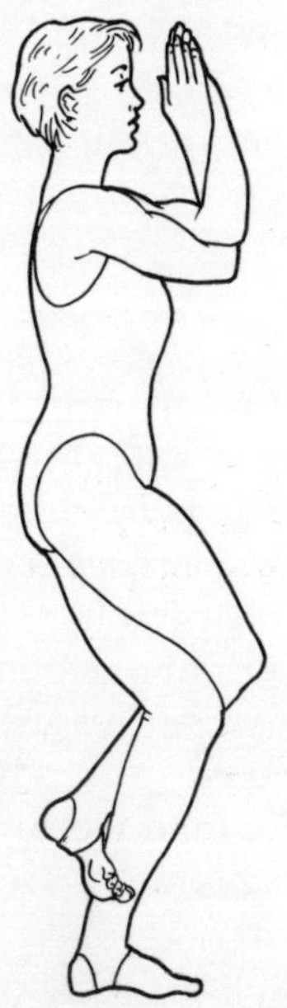

Eagle
The sexual organs are stimulated by the direct pressure on them. The concentration needed to keep your balance is very calming.

Head of a cow
This increases the blood supply to the brain, benefiting the pituitary in particular.

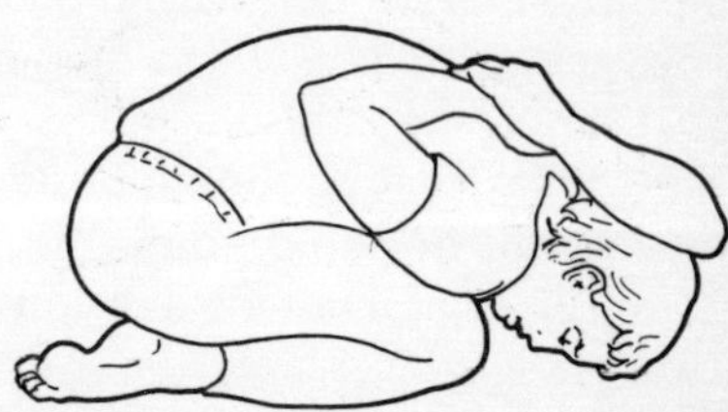

CHAPTER 10

How to find and choose a natural therapist

Tips and guidelines for finding reliable help

It is much easier now to find the right therapist than it was even a few years ago – but it is still not easy enough. The sheer variety of therapies is bewildering in itself and in many countries natural therapists are still not fully organized. There is no shortage of directories and advertisements but it is difficult to know who to rely on for what from lists alone. So how do you find a therapist you can trust?

Starting the search: local sources

As we have seen, many of the natural therapies highlighted in this book have their roots in antiquity. Some have existed for as long as human beings have lived on earth, and finding a good practitioner has been a matter of tuning in to the community 'bush telegraph'. Word of mouth is still the best way to find the right practitioner.

Speak to anyone whose opinion you respect, especially if he or she is also a fellow sufferer. (You will also want to know who should be avoided, and which therapies might not help you at all.) If this does not work there are several other ways you can try.

Doctors' clinics and medical centres

If you need help urgently you must see your family doctor. It has already been explained in this book that your condition can decline quickly without the proper treatment. If you ask about natural therapies at your first appointment, be prepared to hear anything from a dire warning to a recommendation that you might try a natural therapist once your condition is stable.

Natural health centres

Your nearest natural health centre should be happy to advise you. Your first impressions will often be a good guide to the quality of service they provide. Are the staff well informed and friendly? Is the place clean and comfortable? Does the atmosphere make you feel comfortable from the moment you walk in? It should. It matters. You are bringing them your trust and your custom and both should be treated with the utmost respect.

A good centre should have plenty of information explaining the therapies and introducing the practitioners. In a well-run practice the receptionist or owner will know all about the different therapies on offer. It's a bad sign if they don't.

You may still be unsure after your first impressions whether to book in or not. If so, ask to meet the person who might be treating you, just to test the waters. This should be possible, even in a busy practice.

Don't start off by telling your full life history, but some practices do offer you the opportunity of a free consultation – usually 15 minutes – just to see whether you have come to the right place or not.

Local practitioners

Practitioners tend to know who's who in the area, even in therapies other than their own. So if you know, say, a reflexologist, but want a homeopath, ask for a recommendation. The same applies if you know a practitioner socially and so don't want to consult him or her professionally. Practitioners are usually happy to recommend someone else in the same field.

Healthfood stores and alternative bookshops

The staff in these kinds of shops often have a good local knowledge as well as an interest in the subject of natural therapies. The shop may well have a noticeboard with local practitioners' business cards on it. Remember, though, the most experienced and well-established practitioners don't need this kind of advertising, so you might miss them altogether if you don't actually check up by asking.

Other sources of local knowledge

Don't forget that your local pharmacist often has contacts with both conventional and natural therapists.

The local library or information centre may be another good source of contact, especially for finding self-help or support groups.

Computers (using a modem) can provide this type of information via the Internet system and other sources worth trying are health farms, beauty therapists and citizens' advice bureaux.

Wider sources of information

If you have no luck on a local level, don't give up – there are several more leads you can follow up at a national level.

'Umbrella' organizations

The natural therapies are increasingly coming together under 'umbrella' organizations that represent a therapy or range of therapies nationally under one banner or heading. These national umbrella organizations have lists of registered and approved practitioners, and in the case of the more established therapies (such as osteopathy) have their own regulatory bodies already in place.

It is better to phone than to write or fax because this should give you a good idea of how well organized the group is. You may find that the group you are contacting has several different associations under its banner. A small charge may be made for each association's register but if you can afford it get the lot and then make up your own mind.

Newspapers, magazines and local directories

Many therapists advertise. If you find local practitioners this way it's a good idea to talk to them and check them out first.

Checking professional organizations

Some organizations are genuine groups that really keep a check on their members, while others seem to spring up like weeds, apparently interested only in collecting membership fees and giving themselves credibility. This section helps you do your own weeding.

Why do professional organizations exist?

The purposes of governing bodies for natural therapies are:

- to keep up-to-date lists of their members so you can check whether someone is really on their list or not
- to protect you by making sure that their members are fully trained, licensed and insured against accident, negligence and malpractice
- to give you someone to complain to if you are unhappy with any aspect of treatment you have received,

and you can't sort the matter out with your therapist
- to protect their members by giving good ethical and legal advice
- to represent their members when laws which might affect them are being made
- to work towards improvements in education for their members both before and after qualifying
- to work towards greater awareness of the benefit of each therapy in conventional medical circles
- to improve public awareness of the benefit of each therapy

Questions to ask professional organizations

A good organization will publish clear and simple information on its status and purposes along with its membership list. As they don't all do this you may find it useful to contact them again on receiving your list to ask the following questions.

- When was the association founded? (You may be reassured to hear it has been around for 50 years. If the association is new, however, don't reject it out of hand. Ask why it was formed – it may be innovative.)
- How many members does it have? (Size reflects public demand, as few therapists could survive in a therapy if there was no call for it. The bigger organizations generally have a better track record and greater public acceptance, but a small association may just reflect the fact that the therapy is very specialized or still in its infancy – not necessarily a bad thing.)
- When was the therapy that it represents started?
- Is it a charity or educational trust – with a proper constitution, management committee, and published accounts – or is it a private limited company? (Charities have to be non-profitmaking, work in the public interest, and be open to inspection at any time. Private companies don't.)

- Is it part of a larger network of organizations? (If so, this implies it is interested in progress by consensus with other groups, and not just in furthering its own aims. By and large, groups that go their own way are more suspect than those that join in.)
- Does the organization have a code of ethics which upholds standards of professional behaviour and disciplinary procedures? If so, what are they?
- How do its members gain admission to its register? Is it linked to only one school? (Beware of associations whose heads are also head of the school they represent: unbiased help may be in short supply with this type of 'one man band'.)
- Do members have to have proof of professional indemnity insurance? This insurance should cover:
  - accidental damage to yourself or your property while you are on the practitioner's work premises
  - negligence (either the failure of the practitioner to exercise the 'duty of care' owed to you, or his falling below the standards of clinical competence demand ed by his qualifications, bringing about an overall worsening of your problem)
  - malpractice (a 'falling from grace' over professional conduct, involving, for example, dishonesty, sexual misconduct or breach of confidence – your personal details should *never* be discussed with a third person without your permission)

Checking training and qualifications

If you have reassured yourself so far but are still puzzled by what the training actually involves, ask a few more questions.

- How long is the training?
- Is it full or part time?
- If it is part-time but shorter than a full-time course

leading to the same qualifications, does the time spent at lectures and in clinic add up to the same as a full-time course overall? (In other words, is it a short cut?)
- Does it include seeing patients under supervision at a college clinic and in real practices?
- What do the initials after the therapist's name mean? Do they denote simply membership of an organization or do they indicate in-depth study?
- Are the qualifications recognized? If so, by whom? (This is becoming more relevant as the therapy organizations group together and form state-recognized registers in many countries. But the really important thing to know is if the qualifications are recognized by an independent outside assessment authority.)

Making the choice

Making the final choice is a matter of using your common sense and intuition, and finding the resolution to give someone a try. Don't forget that the most important part of the whole process is your resolve to feel better, to have more control over your state of health, and to see an improvement in your condition. The next most important part is that you feel comfortable with your chosen therapist.

What is it like seeing a natural therapist?

Since most natural therapists, even in those countries with state health systems, still work privately, there is no established common pattern.

Although they may all share more or less a belief in the principles outlined in Chapter 6, you are liable to come across individuals from all walks of life. You will find as much variety in dress, thinking and behaviour as there are fashions, ranging from the formal and sophisticated to the absolutely informal.

Equally, you will find their premises very different. Some will present a 'brass plaque' image, working in a clinic with a receptionist and brisk efficiency, while others will see you in their living room surrounded by plants and domestic clutter.

Remember, though, that while image may be some indication of status, it is little guarantee of ability. You are as likely to find a therapist of quality working from home as in a formal clinic.

Some characteristics, though, and probably the most important ones, are common to all natural therapists.

- They will give you far more time than you are used to with a family doctor. An initial consultation will rarely last less than an hour, and is often longer. They will ask you all about yourself so they can form a proper understanding of what makes you tick and what may be the fundamental cause(s) of your problem.
- You will have to pay for any remedies they prescribe, and they may well sell you these from their own stocks. They will also charge you for their time – though many therapists offer reduced fees for deserving cases or for people who genuinely cannot afford the full fee.

Sensible precautions

- Be sceptical of anyone who 'guarantees' you a cure. No-one (not even doctors) can do that.
- Query any attempt to book you in for a course of treatment. Your response to any natural therapy is highly individual. Of course, if the practice is a busy one, booking ahead for one or two sessions might be sensible. You should be able to cancel without penalty any

sessions which prove unnecessary (but remember to give at least 24 hours' notice: some practitioners will charge you if you don't give enough notice).

- No ethical therapist will ask for fees in advance of treatment unless for special tests or medicines – and even this is unusual. If you are asked for 'down payments' of any sort, ask exactly what they are for. If you don't like the reasons, don't pay.
- Be wary if you are not asked about your existing medication and try to give precise answers when you are asked. Be especially wary if the therapist tells you to stop or change any medically prescribed drug without talking to your doctor first. (A responsible doctor should also be happy to discuss you and your medication with a therapist.)
- Note the quality of the therapist's touch if you choose any of the relaxation or manipulation techniques such as massage, aromatherapy or osteopathy. It should never be lingering or suggestive. If, for any reason, the therapist wants to touch you on the breasts or genitals, your permission should be sought first.
- If the practitioner is of the opposite sex you are entitled to have someone of your choice in the room at the same time. Be immediately suspicious if this is not allowed. Ethical therapists will not refuse this sort of request, and if they do, it is probably best to have nothing more to do with them.

What to do if things go wrong

A practitioner is in a position of trust, and is charged with a duty of care to you at all times. It does not mean you are 'entitled' to a 'cure' just because you've paid for treatment, but if you feel you are being treated unfairly, incompetently or unethically, you have several options.

- Tackle the matter at the source of the problem, with your practitioner, either verbally or in writing.
- If he or she works in a place such as a clinic, health farm or sports centre, tell the management. They also have a duty to protect the public and should treat complaints seriously and discreetly.
- Contact the practitioner's professional organization. It should have an independent panel that investigates complaints fully and disciplines its members.
- If the offence committed is a criminal one report it to the police (but be prepared for the problem of proving one person's word against another's).
- If you feel compensation is due see a lawyer for advice.

Short of a public court case, the worst thing for a truly incompetent or unethical practitioner is bad publicity. Tell everyone about your experiences. People only need to hear the same sort of comments from a few different sources and the practitioner will probably sink without trace. Before you do so, though, try the other measures first and give yourself time to consider things calmly. Vengeance is not very healing.

A word of warning Don't make malicious allegations without good reason. Such actions are themselves a criminal offence in most countries and you could end up in more trouble than the practitioner.

Summary

The reality is that there are few real crooks or charlatans in natural therapy. Despite the myth, there is little real money in it unless the therapist is very busy – and the chances are high that a busy therapist is a good one. Remember that no-one can know everything and no specialist qualified in any field has to get 100 per cent in the exams to be able to practise. Perfection is an ideal, not a reality, and to err is human.

It is very much for this reason that taking control of your own health is perhaps the single most important lesson underlying this book. Taking control means taking responsibility for the choices you make, and this is one of the most significant factors in successful treatment.

No-one but you can decide on a practitioner and no-one but you can determine if that practitioner is any good or not. You will know this very easily, and probably very quickly, by the way you feel about the person and the therapy, and by whether or not you get any better.

If you are not happy, the decision is yours whether to stay or move on – and continue moving until you find the right therapist for you. Don't despair if you don't find the right person first time. There is almost bound to be the right person for you somewhere and your determination to get well is the best resource you have for finding that person.

Above all, bear in mind that many people who have taken this route before you have not only been helped beyond their most optimistic dreams, but have also found a close and trusted helper who will assist in times of trouble – and who may even become a friend for life.

APPENDIX A

Glossary of acronyms

AID	artificial insemination by donor (same as DI)
AIH/P	artificial insemination by husband/partner
BBT	basal body temperature
DI	donor insemination (same as AID)
EFA	essential fatty acid
FSH	follicle stimulating hormone
GIFT	gamete intra fallopian transfer
GNRH	gonadotrophin releasing hormone
GU	genito-urinary
HCG	human chorionic gonadotrophin
HFEA	Human Fertilization and Embryology Authority
HMG	human menopausal gonadotrophin
HRT	hormone replacement therapy
HSG	hysterosalpingogram/phy
ICSI	intra cytoplasmic sperm injection
IU(C)D	intra uterine (contraceptive) device
IUI	intra uterine insemination
IVF	in vitro fertilization
LH	luteinizing hormone
LHRH	LH releasing hormone
LOD	ovarian diathermy by laparoscopy
MAF	micro assisted fertilization
MESA	micro epididymal sperm aspiration
OHSS	ovarian hyper-stimulation syndrome
PCB	polychlorinatedbiphenyl
PCOD/S	polycystic ovary disease/syndrome
PCT	post-coital test
PID	pelvic inflammatory disease
PROST	pronuclear stage tubal transfer (same as ZIFT)
PZD	partial zonal dissection
RDA	recommended daily amount (of vitamins and minerals)
STD	sexually transmitted disease

SUZI	sub zonal insemination
TCM	Traditional Chinese Medicine
UDOR	ultrasound-directed oocyte recovery
ZIFT	zygote intra fallopian transfer (same as PROST)

APPENDIX B

Useful organizations

The following listing of organizations is for information only and does not imply any endorsement, nor do the organizations listed necessarily agree with the views expressed in this book.

INTERNATIONAL

International Federation of Practitioners of Natural Therapeutics
10 Copse Close
Sheet, Petersfield
Hampshire GU31 4DL
UK.
Tel 01730 266790
Fax 01730 260058

AUSTRALIA

Australian Natural Therapists Association
PO Box 308
Melrose Park
South Australia 5039.
Tel 8297 9533
Fax 8297 0003

Australian Traditional Medicine Society
PO Box 442
Suite 3, First Floor
120 Blaxland Road
Ryde, NSW 2112.
Tel 2808 2825
Fax 2809 7570

Family Planning Federation of Australia
24 Campbell Street
Sydney, NSW 2000.

Foresight
Mrs P Quinn
124 Louisa Road
Birchgrove, NSW.

OASIS
Infertility Support Group
GPO Box 2420
Adelaide 5001
South Australia.

NEW ZEALAND

Auckland Infertility Society
PO Box 68428
Auckland.

Christchurch Infertility Society
PO Box 29188
Christchurch.

Fertility Action
PO Box 4569/
2nd Floor, 27 Gillies Avenue
Newmarket
Auckland 1.
Tel 9520 5295

New Zealand Family Planning Association
PO Box 68-200/
214 Karangahape Road
Auckland 1.

New Zealand Natural Health Practitioners Accreditation Board
PO Box 37-491
Auckland.
Tel 9625 9966

Otago/Southland Infertility Society
PO Box 6286
Dunedin North.

Wellington Infertility Society
PO Box 31279
Lower Hutt.

Womanline
Women's Health Centre
63 Ponsonby Road
Auckland.
Tel 9376 5173

NORTH AMERICA

American Association of Naturopathic Physicians
2800 East Madison Street
Suite 200, Seattle
Washington 98112, USA
or
PO Box 20386
Seattle
Washington 98102, USA.
Tel 206 323 7610
Fax 206 323 7612

American Holistic Medical Association
6728 Old McLean Village Drive
McLean, VA 22101, USA
Tel 703 556 9222

Canadian Holistic Medical Association
700 Bay Street
PO Box 101, Suite 604
Toronto
Ontario M5G 1Z6, Canada.
Tel 416 599 0447

Flower Essence Society
PO Box 1769
Nevada City
California 95959, USA.
Tel 916 265 9163/0258
Fax 916 265 6467
Information on flower remedies

Foresight
Mr Richard Piccolo
4223 Sunney-Side Drive
RD 4 Doylestown
Pennsylvania 18901, USA.

SOUTH AFRICA

Foresight
Mrs C Raciborska
3 Ireland Road
Oak Park
Pietermaritzburg
Natal 3201, RSA

South Africa Homeopaths, Chiropractors and Allied Professions Board
PO Box 17055
0027 Groenkloof
Transvaal, RSA.
Tel 2712 466 455

UK

British Complementary Medicine Association
39 Prestbury Road
Pitville
Cheltenham
Glos GL52 2PT.
Tel 01242 226770
Fax 01242 226778

British Holistic Medical Association
Royal Shrewsbury Hospital South
Shrewsbury
Shropshire SY3 8XF.
Tel 01743 261155
Fax 01743 353637

CHILD
Charter House
43 St Leonards Road
Bexhill on Sea
East Sussex TN40 1JA.
Tel 01424 732361
Fax 01424 731858
Support group for those undergoing conventional treatment

Council for Complementary and Alternative Medicine
Park House
206-208 Latimer Road
London W10 6RE.
Tel 0181 968 3862
Fax 0181 968 3469

Dr Edward Bach Centre
Mount Vernon
Sotwell
Wallingford
Oxfordshire OX10 0PZ.
Tel 01491 834678
Fax 01491 825022
Advice and information about Bach Flower Remedies

Foresight
28 The Paddock
Godalming
Surrey GU7 1XD.
Tel 01483 427839
Information on infertility self-help and preconception care

Human Fertilization and Embryology Authority
Paxton House
30 Artillery Lane
London E1 7LS.
Tel 0171 377 5077
Fax 0171 377 1871
Information on assisted conception techniques and the law relating to them, and on choosing a clinic

Institute for Complementary Medicine
PO Box 194
London SE16 1QZ.
Tel 0171 237 5165
Fax 0171 237 5175

ISSUE (National Fertility Association)
509 Aldridge Road
Great Barr
Birmingham B44 8NA.
Tel 0121 344 4414
Fax 0121 344 4336
Medical advice, counselling and local support groups

National Infertility Awareness Campaign
99 Bridge Road East
Welwyn Garden City
Hertfordshire AL7 1BG.
Information on the availability of conventional treatment in different parts of the country

Natural Family Planning Centre
Queen Elizabeth Medical Centre
Birmingham.
Tel 0121 472 1377 ext 4219
or
Mrs Colleen Norman
218 Heathwood Road
Heath
Cardiff CF4 4BS.
Tel 01222 754628
For list of natural family planning teachers

Soil Association
86 Colston Street
Bristol BS1 5BB
Tel 0117 929 0661
Information on where to buy organic food

EIRE

Foresight
Mrs P Quinn
Sunneyhill
Bohernabrena
Dublin 24

APPENDIX C

Useful further reading and listening

Books

Acupuncture, Peter Mole (Element, UK, USA and Australia, 1992)

Aromatherapy, Christine Wildwood (Element, UK, USA and Australia, 1991)

Art of Shiatsu, Oliver Cowmeadow (Element, UK, USA and Australia, 1992)

Bach Flower Remedies for Women, Judy Howard (C W Daniel, UK, 1992)

Complete Hatha Yoga, Kevin and Venika Kingsland (Arco, USA, 1983)

Getting Pregnant: The complete guide to fertility and infertility Prof Robert Winston (Pan, UK, 1993)

Hypnosis, Ursula Markham (Macdonald Optima, UK, 1987)

Infertility: A common-sense guide for the childless (also called *Why Us?*), Dr Andrew Stanway (Thorsons, UK, 1984)

Infertility: Your questions answered Seang Lin Tan and Howard Jacobs (McGraw-Hill, Singapore, USA, NZ, UK, Canada and Australia, 1991)

Is Acupuncture for You?, J R Worsley (Element, UK, USA and Australia, 1985)

Reader's Digest Family Guide to Alternative Medicine (The Reader's Digest Association, UK, USA, Australia, Canada, S Africa, 1991)

Research in Healing, Dan Benor (Helix, Germany and UK, 1994)

The Elements of Meditation, David Fontana (Element, UK, USA and Australia 1991)

The Experience of Infertility, Naomi Pfeffer and Anne Woollett (Virago, UK, 1983)

The Fertility and Contraception Book, Julia Mosse and Josephine Heaton (Faber and Faber, UK and US, 1990)

Tapes

Self-hypnosis cassettes for infertility and relaxation or made specially for you from:

Pilgrim Tapes
PO Box 107
Shrewsbury SY1 1ZZ, UK.

Tapes for Health
British Holistic Medical Association
Shrewsbury SY3 8XF, UK.

Index

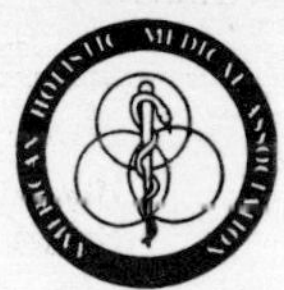

BHMA TAPES FOR HEALTH

Practical self-help packages designed by experts to make taking care of yourself easier

Imagery For Relaxation by Duncan Johnson
Exercises in visualization to help relaxation and influence the functions of the body and mind. To provide yourself with the opportunity to learn more about your attitudes and neglected needs. To harness the forces of the creative mind and change negative attitudes to life.

Getting To Sleep by Ashley Conway
A practical help with insomnia. Promotes relaxation and positive thinking to put you in touch with your body's 'normal' sleep pattern.

Introduction To Meditation by Dr Sarah Eagger
This tape is a progressive learning programme of meditation exercises. Teaching you how to begin using meditation for increasing your peace of mind and well-being.

Coping With Persistent Pain by Dr James Hawkins
Teaches relaxation skills in a greater depth, and how to apply those skills as a coping method during daily activities. To help promote some form of normality into a life of constant pain.

Coping With Stress by Dr David Peters
A programme to teach you how to build the relaxation response into your life. Understanding stress and dealing with it through relaxation techniques.

The Breath Of Life by Dr Patrick Pietroni
A muscular relaxation technique which explores the connection between stress and our breathing rhythm. With exercises on how to control breathing to alleviate symptoms of stress.

Please write to the British Holistic Medical Association at Rowland Thomas House, Royal Shrewsbury Hospital South, Shrewsbury, Shropshire, SY3 8XF for full details of tapes and mail order service.